Perioperative Drill-Based Crisis Management

Perioperative Drill-Based Crisis Management

Edited by

Steven Butz
Medical College of Wisconsin, Milwaukee, WI, USA

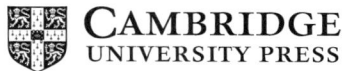

CAMBRIDGE
UNIVERSITY PRESS

University Printing House, Cambridge CB2 8BS, United Kingdom

Cambridge University Press is part of the University of Cambridge.

It furthers the University's mission by disseminating knowledge in the pursuit of
education, learning and research at the highest international levels of excellence.

www.cambridge.org
Information on this title: www.cambridge.org/9781107546936

First published 2016

Printed in the United Kingdom by TJ International Ltd. Padstow Cornwall

A catalogue record for this publication is available from the British Library

Library of Congress Cataloguing in Publication data
Perioperative drill-based crisis management / edited by Steven Butz.
     p.   ;   cm.
Includes bibliographical references and index.
ISBN 978-1-107-54693-6 (paperback)
I. Butz, Steven, 1967–, editor.
[DNLM: 1. Perioperative Care.   2. Ambulatory Care Facilities–organization & administration.
3. Intraoperative Complications–prevention & control.   4. Patient Simulation.   5. Safety Management–
organization & administration.   6. Workplace Violence–prevention & control. WO 178]
RA974
362.12–dc23   2015023051

ISBN 978-1-107-54693-6 Paperback

Contents

Contributors

Claude Abdallah, MD, MSc
Children's National Health System, Division of
Anesthesiology, Sedation and Perioperative Medicine,
Washington DC, USA

Fatima Ahmad, MD
Associate Professor at the Department of
Anesthesiology, Loyola University Chicago,
Chicago, IL, USA

Shyamal Asher, MD
Resident Physician, Department of Anesthesia and
Critical Care, University of Chicago, Chicago, IL, USA

Steven Butz, MD
Associate Professor of Anesthesiology at the Medical
College of Wisconsin, Milwaukee, and Medical
Director at the Children's Hospital of Wisconsin
Surgicenter, Milwaukee, WI, USA

Rose Campise-Luther, MD, FAAP
Children's Hospital of Wisconsin and Medical College
of Wisconsin, WI, USA

David M. Dickerson, MD
Assistant Professor at the Department of Anesthesia
and Critical Care, University of Chicago, Chicago,
IL, USA

Deborah S. Lowery, MD
Clinical Assistant Professor of Anesthesiology at The
Eye and Ear Institute Outpatient Surgery Center,
The Ohio State University Wexner Medical Center,
Columbus, OH, USA

Niraja Rajan, MD
Medical Director at the Hershey Outpatient Surgery
Center and Assistant Professor of Anesthesiology
at the Penn State Hershey Medical Center, Hershey,
PA, USA

Catherine Schulz, MD
Assistant Professor of Clinical Anesthesiology and
Director of Resident Simulation Education, University
of Southern California Keck School of Medicine, Los
Angeles, CA, USA

Amir Shbeeb, MD
Resident Physician, LAC+USC Medical Center,
Department of Anesthesiology, Los Angeles,
CA, USA

Connie K. Tran, MD
Associate Professor and Co-Director, Acute
Pain Management Service at the Department of
Anesthesiology, and Mentor, BCM Student
Mentoring Program at the Baylor College of
Medicine, Houston, TX, USA

Sonal N. Zambare, MD
Fellow, Obstetric Anesthesiology Department of
Anesthesiology, Baylor College of Medicine, Houston,
TX, USA

Preface

This manual was developed to help medical directors and administrators run drills at their healthcare facilities. Although this was primarily designed with ambulatory surgical facilities in mind, it can be used by hospitals and office settings where patient care takes place. The chapters will lead a person through a drill. The drill unfolds stepwise and will be broken up with actions that the participants are expected to take. This will help the drill instructor to lead the participants down a particular pathway if they start to "wander".

The chapters are organized by group. The first two are general enough to be used by any facility. The stems are surgical, but can be generalized to any patient population. Chapters 3 to 8 are surgery specific. They deal with health issues that are unique to the surgical setting. The last two chapters are applicable to any setting. The book is written from a surgical point of view, but really applies to any building that is open to the public.

The layout of each chapter is consistent. There is an introduction with learning goals. Drill scenarios follow that flow between an evolving story and what anticipated actions are. There are at least three drills per chapter. Following the scenarios are debriefing questions and then the detailed discussion with learning points. This permits any drill leader to be an "expert" even if addressing a scenario outside his or her field of expertise. If a group of scenarios is closely related, the debriefing will follow after the last scenario. If the scenarios are very individual, the debrief and discussion unique to each case will follow immediately.

As stated, the drills can be used "out of the box", but there are some tips to make them work better. First of all, the person running the drill should read the entire drill, debrief and discussion. This will help focus the drill and bring up relevant questions. When doing a drill myself and I see that the staff is on a tangent or not able to pick up correctly on the problem I am presenting, I will have an imaginary colleague "stop by" and give advice. I may say, "Another anesthesiologist steps in and says that the last time he saw a patient not wake up, we checked his blood sugar." That way the drill can continue in the direction intended and people accept it as part of the drill without taking offense like they are doing something wrong.

In much the same way, a scenario stem can be changed to fit a different setting. Instead of a patient having crushing chest pain in the recovery room, they can present to the front desk of a medical office or urgent care. The rest of the story can be easily tailored from there.

Medical lingo has many acronyms and regional abbreviations. Many of these were edited out, but a glossary was also put in to help. Sometimes a term is defined early in the chapter, but may appear again in the drill. This may confuse someone that hasn't heard it before. All abbreviations and some geographically regional terms are all placed alphabetically in the glossary. As an additional note, this American-written book uses lab values common in the United States. For instance, blood sugars are reported in mg/dl and partial pressures are in mmHg. A book that contains algorithms for ACLS will make a great companion to this book. Many of these are widely available and are of great quality. Most common are the products of the American Heart Association for Advanced Cardiac Life Support or Pediatric Advanced Life Support.

I hope people learn as much from using this book as I did writing and editing it. Most of all, I hope that it increases the quality and quantity of drills performed by a medical team and all with less effort!

Glossary of terms

"9-1-1" or "911"	Emergency number in United States that connects to a municipality's joint answering center for police, ambulance or fire emergencies
"9/11"	Refers to bombing incident on Sept 11, 2001 when terrorists piloted jet liners into the World Trade Center in New York City and the Pentagon in Washington, DC. A fourth plane was downed by passengers in Pennsylvania
AA	Anesthesia Assistant; a physician assistant specialty trained in anesthesia
A-a gradient	Difference between alveolar and arterial concentrations, most commonly in reference to oxygen levels
ABG	Arterial blood gas
ACL	Anterior cruciate ligament
ACLS	Advanced Cardiac Life Support, an American Heart Association course that teaches pathways or algorithms using drugs and defibrillation/pacing to treat many causes of cardiac arrest, shock and stroke
ACS	Acute coronary syndrome
AED	Automated external defibrillator
AFOI	Awake fiberoptic intubation
AMBU	Artificial manual breathing unit
ASA	American Society of Anesthesiologists
ASC	Ambulatory surgery center, usually freestanding and completely separated from a hospital
ASRA	American Society of Regional Anesthesia
ATP	Adenosine triphosphate
BLS	Basic life support which is essentially chest compressions and rescue breathing without administering drugs
BMI	Body Mass Index; developed to quantify obesity by more than just weight. May be elevated for a very muscular individual. The calculation is weight (kg)/height (m) squared
Cath	Short for catheter or catheterization as in a cardiac catheterization laboratory or suite
CKD	Chronic kidney disease
CK-MB	Creatine kinase enzyme with myocardial subtype indicative of myocardial infarction when released into the bloodstream and measurable via a laboratory serum test
CMS	Centers for Medicare and Medicaid Services; a US agency that acts as a national health insurance for the poor and elderly. It creates many conditions to participate in caring for its patients that are, in effect, federal law
CNS	Central nervous system, i.e. brain and spinal cord
CPAP	Continuous positive airway pressure
CPR	Cardiopulmonary resuscitation
Crash cart	Rolling cart that is typically stocked with resuscitation drugs and equipment necessary to run a cardiac resuscitation
CRNA	Certified Registered Nurse Anesthetist
DC	Direct current

DKA	Diabetic ketoacidosis
EAP	Emergency action plan
ECG/EKG	Electrocardiogram
EF	Ejection fraction, specifically cardiac
EMS	Emergency medical services, typically a transport ambulance staffed with paramedics or emergency medical technicians
ENT	Otolaryngology or "Ears, Nose and Throat" specialists
ETT	Endotracheal tube
FBI	Federal Bureau of Investigation; a police force in the United States with the entire country as its jurisdiction
FEMA	Federal Emergency Management Agency; a US agency that manages disasters (natural or man-made) within the US borders
FiO_2	Fraction of inspired air that is oxygen
GERD	Gastroesophageal reflux disease
GETA	General endotracheal anesthesia; a general anesthetic using an endotracheal tube as an airway
HAZMAT	Hazardous material
HR	Heart rate
HTN	Arterial hypertension or high blood pressure
HVAC	Heating, ventilation, air-conditioning; a building's heating and cooling system
IC	Incident commander
ICU	Intensive Care Unit; critical care unit with ability to have patients on ventilators, vasoactive drips, and invasive monitoring
IED	Improvised incendiary or explosive device
ILCOR	International Liaison Committee on Resuscitation
IT	Information technology; a facility's computer system
IV	Intravenous, as in intravenous route of medicine administration or as in a peripheral intravenous line
JVD	Jugular venous distension
LAD	Left anterior descending coronary artery
LAST	Local anesthetic systemic toxicity
LMA	Laryngeal mask airway specifically, or any supraglottic airway in general terms
LR	Lactated Ringer's, a balanced intravenous fluid solution
LVH	Left ventricular hypertrophy
MAC	Monitored anesthesia care; a billing term, but used to indicate procedural sedation given by an anesthesia provider
MH	Malignant hyperthermia
MHAUS	Malignant Hyperthermia Association of the United States. They run the 24-hour MH hotline, 800-644-9737, staffed full-time by MH experts
MI	Myocardial infarct or heart attack
min	Minute
NIBP	Non-invasive blood pressure
NIDDM	Non-insulin dependent diabetes mellitus
NPO	Nil per os; fasting
NSAID	Non-steroidal anti-inflammatory drug
ORIF	Open reduction internal fixation
$PaCO_2$	Partial pressure of arterial carbon dioxide
PACU	Post-Anesthesia Care Unit, generally the area in which patients first recover from a general anesthetic
PCA	Post-conceptual age; the estimation of the number of weeks of age from conception for a fetus or infant

PCI	Percutaneous cardiac intervention
PE	Pulmonary embolism
PEA	Pulseless electrical activity
PEEP	Positive end expiratory pressure
PPV	Positive pressure ventilation
PR	Electrocardiogram segment from the P-wave to the R-wave
PTT/ptt	Partial thromboplastin time; a measure of heparin effectiveness on a patient
PVC	Premature ventricular contraction
QRS	The waves on an electocardiogram that reflect ventricular contraction
QT	Electrocardiogram segment from the Q-wave to the T-wave
RCA	Right coronary artery
Remorphinization	When an opioid is reversed by naloxone, there is a risk that the shorter half-life of naloxone will allow it to wear off while a significant amount of morphine (opioid) is still present and sedation and hypoventilation may recur
SGA	Supraglottic airway
s/p	Status post
SpO_2	Oxygen saturation from a pulse oximeter reading
ST	The segment on an electrocardiogram between the S- and T-waves
STEMI	ST-segment elevation myocardial infarction
SVR	Systemic vascular resistance
TEE	Trans-esophogeal echocardiography
TIVA	Total intravenous anesthetic, as in no inhalational component
TOF	Train of four
VF	Ventricular fibrillation
VT	Ventricular tachycardia
VTE	Venous thromboembolism

Cardiac arrest
Acute coronary syndrome

Amir Shbeeb and Catherine Schulz

Introduction

Cardiac arrest is a rare but serious cause of morbidity and mortality in the perioperative setting. Ischemic heart disease is the leading cause of death in the world.[1] Ambulatory surgery centers should be prepared to treat acute coronary syndrome (ACS) and have a system in place to stabilize and transfer the patient to a higher acuity level of care facility, and if possible one that has a cardiac catheterization lab. The principles in this case apply to any operating room (hospital-based and outpatient), off-site anesthetizing location, or clinic.

The three cases presented here for learning purposes are patients with preexisting coronary artery disease presenting for elective ambulatory surgery. Theses cases will offer an opportunity to discuss key points in early detection, communication, treatment, and management.

Educational objectives

1. Take appropriate steps to manage a patient with known or possible coronary artery disease
2. Detect early signs of myocardial ischemia or cardiac arrest
3. Emergently treat cardiac arrest

Scenario 1: STEMI in operating room

A 76-year-old male, 82 kg patient is in the operating room for a shoulder arthroscopy. The patient has a history of hypertension, hyperlipidemia, coronary artery disease, and diabetes mellitus type 2, all of which are moderately well controlled with medications. General anesthesia induction was uneventful. During surgical incision, tachycardia and ST segment elevation in leads II and V5 were detected.

Expected actions:

1. Assess clinical status and check all vital signs
2. Assure ventilation and oxygenation
3. Consider early treatment prior to confirming diagnosis

Scenario continued:

Acute hypotension quickly ensues with decrease in end-tidal CO_2.

Expected actions:

1. Call for help and ask for crash cart
2. Consider placing invasive arterial line
3. Check blood pressure and other vital signs
4. Differential diagnosis of acute myocardial infarction, pulmonary embolus, anaphylaxis, hypovolemia
5. Consider placement of trans-esophageal echo probe (TEE) for diagnosis (if available)

Scenario continued:

TEE reveals anteroseptal and inferior wall hypokinesis. (If no TEE available, downsloping ST-segments are seen on anterior and inferior leads of 12-lead ECG.)

Expected actions:

1. Consider acute myocardial ischemia causes: coronary artery spasm, plaque rupture, demand ischemia
2. Begin vasodilator and inotrope infusion as needed to maintain blood pressure (nitroglycerin and epinephrine)

Perioperative Drill-Based Crisis Management, ed. Steven Butz. Published by Cambridge University Press. © Cambridge University Press 2016.

Scenario continued:

Ventricular ectopy, deteriorates into ventricular fibrillation

Expected actions:

1. Begin basic life support (BLS). This is chest compressions at ratio of 30 compressions to two breaths, rate at least 100, depth at least 2" (5 cm), allow for recoil
2. Get defibrillator and attach pads
3. Simultaneously secure airway depending on expertise of available staff (mask ventilate, supraglottic airway, or intubation)
4. Defibrillate at 200 joules, repeat after 2 min at 360 if unsuccessful

Scenario continued:

Rhythm converts to sinus rhythm with occasional PVCs, blood pressure 98/74, HR 88

Expected actions:

1. Continue treatment with fluids and vasoactive medications
2. Continue to monitor vital signs and echo imaging
3. Arrange disposition to higher level of care facility with cardiac catheterization lab capabilities

The drill ends with resuscitation that continues in transport to hospital with cardiac catheterization lab.

Scenario 2: Chest pain in recovery

A 77-year-old female 67 kg patient is in the post anesthesia care unit (PACU) recovering from a carpal tunnel release under local anesthesia with monitored anesthesia care. She has a history of chronic kidney disease (CKD) requiring dialysis, hypertension, diabetes mellitus type 2, and coronary artery disease. She had suffered a heart attack 12 months previously, requiring two stents in her proximal LAD and one in the mid RCA. The MI was complicated by heart failure with an EF of 24% requiring an aortic balloon pump, but she has regained some functional capacity walking two blocks slowly. The patient begins to complain of severe crushing substernal chest pain upon arrival in PACU and calls out to her nurse.

Expected actions:

1. Call for help and ask for crash cart
2. Obtain 12-lead ECG

3. Administer oxygen via nasal cannula, increase as needed to maintain oxygen saturation greater than 90%
4. Administer chewable aspirin 162–325 mg non enteric coated
5. Give sublingual nitroglycerin as needed for chest pain
6. Administer morphine intravenously as needed for chest pain
7. Consider differential diagnosis including aortic dissection, pericarditis, pulmonary embolus, pneumonia, pneumothorax, pleuritis, gastrointestinal reflux disease, esophageal spasm, costochondritis, etc.

Scenario continued:

ST elevation is noted in the anterior leads V1–V4, ventricular ectopy begins, and the cardiac rhythm rapidly deteriorates to ventricular fibrillation

Expected actions:

1. Begin basic life support
2. Get defibrillator and attach pads
3. Simultaneously secure airway depending on expertise of available staff (mask ventilate, supraglottic airway or intubation)
4. Defibrillate at 200 joules, repeat after 2 min at 360 if unsuccessful

Scenario continued:

Defibrillation success, patient is stable, blood pressure is 94/62, HR 85.

Expected actions:

1. If freestanding center, call EMS for transfer using pre-established institutional management protocols of STEMI
2. If tertiary care center, institute single call system for mobilization to cardiac catheter lab with cardiology consult for angiography
3. Establish arterial line and send labs for multimarker evaluation with cardiac troponin and creatine kinase MB (CK-MB)
4. Support circulation with inotropes and antiarrhythmic as necessary

Scenario continued:

The drill ends with implementation of protocol to transfer patient to facility with cath lab alerted to possible acute stent thrombosis.

Scenario 3: Bradycardic arrest

A 59-year-old male is in the operating room receiving a retrobulbar block by the ophthalmologist for a planned vitrectomy. He has a past medical history of diabetes mellitus type 2, HTN, sleep apnea, and hyperlipidemia. After injection of 3 ml of lidocaine 2% mixed with bupivacaine 0.75% the patient becomes severely bradycardic to a rate of <20. The patient is given glycopyrrolate 0.2 mg IV with no response and subsequently is given atropine 0.4 mg IV. The patient then responds with sinus tachycardia at a rate of 142 and begins to complain of chest pain.

Expected actions:

1. Treat tachycardia with beta-blocker
2. Administer O_2 via nasal cannula to keep saturation greater than 90%
3. Obtain 12-lead ECG
4. Obtain serial cardiac troponin levels (at presentation and at 3 and 6 hours)
5. Review medical history and reassess risk

Scenario continued:

A 12-lead ECG reveals down-sloping ST depression and T-wave inversion anteriorly. Patient continues complaining of symptoms of chest tightness and inability to breathe. Patient becomes diaphoretic. Heart rate decreases to 90 but chest pain continues.

Expected actions:

1. Administer sublingual nitroglycerin 0.4 mg every 5 min up to three doses (contraindicated if patient on phosphodiesterase inhibitor)
2. Give intravenous morphine for pain
3. Administer chewable aspirin 162–325 mg non enteric coated
4. Call for help for cardiac evaluation if available
5. Consider use of oral beta-blockers, calcium channel blockers, and statins

Scenario continued:

Drill ends with making urgent arrangements to transfer patient to cardiac care unit or another facility because of ongoing chest pain.

Debriefing

Briefings happen before a learning experience, and debriefings after. Debriefing is a form of feedback, and allows the participants to reflect on their knowledge and behavioral and technical skills. It is important to have the participants feel safe to question and not take the feedback as a personal attack, but to welcome the opportunity to find their own knowledge gaps and or discover themselves what they needed to do better. That is the art of debriefing. The participants should feel empowered to recognize themselves their own strengths and weaknesses. It is thought that this active learning enhances memory.

1. Identify three things the team felt went well during the scenario.
2. Identify three things the team felt should or could be improved.
3. What equipment was difficult to locate or use?
4. Was crash cart or TEE probe difficult to obtain?
5. Was help easily accessible?
6. What was not available that would have been helpful?
7. What would have been done differently?
8. Discuss when you thought transfer to hospital with or without cardiac catheterization lab would be necessary.
9. Discuss the steps of ACLS resuscitation and algorithm.
10. Identify up to three improvements that the facility will incorporate after the drill to prepare them for a similar case.

Discussion

The American College of Cardiology (ACC) and American Heart Association (AHA) provided updated guidelines for risk assessment of non-cardiac surgery and need for perioperative workup and management.[2] The ACC & AHA have also provided updated recommendations for management of acute coronary syndrome.[3,4] The underlying principle for their recommendations is to use appropriate key clinical factors such as type of surgery and patient comorbidities to assess risk, which guides the degree of preoperative cardiac workup for non-cardiac surgery. For patients experiencing acute coronary syndrome, efficient teamwork is essential in stabilizing patient transfer to a hospital with cardiac catheterization lab capabilities.

Initial medical therapy should consist of immediate antiplatelet anticoagulant therapy. Despite the proliferation of newer antiplatelet and antithrombotic agents, aspirin continues to be the mainstay of initial management and should not be forgotten. Oxygen, nitrates, beta-blockers, calcium channel blockers, and statins are Class I therapy (benefit is greater than risk, procedure/treatment should be performed/administered). Morphine sulfate is reasonable for treatment of continued pain despite maximal medical therapy, even though it is classified as a type IIb agent (benefit greater or equal to risk, additional studies needed. Procedure treatment may be considered).[3]

Nitrates in the setting of phosphodiesterase therapy, NSAIDS, IV beta-blockers when shock is present, and immediate-release nifedipine in the absence of a beta-blocker are all potentially harmful interventions in acute coronary syndrome.[3]

The International Liaison Committee on Resuscitation (ILCOR) includes representatives from the AHA, the European Resuscitation Council (ERC), the Heart and Stroke Foundation of Canada (HSFC), the Australian and New Zealand Committee on Resuscitation (ANZCOR), and the Resuscitation Council of Asia (RCA). They have established an updated ILCOR Universal Cardiac Arrest Algorithm,[1] which has only two pathways, shockable or non-shockable cardiac rhythm. These documents are available on the ILCOR website (see www.ilcor.org). A simple algorithm to follow has the benefit of allowing the staff to focus on the quality of the CPR efforts and early defibrillation, which has been shown to improve outcomes.

Early recognition of myocardial ischemia is the key to management, along with having existing protocols and systems in place for handling emergencies. In an effort to do no harm, medical professionals may have a tendency toward inaction rather than action, and avoid starting CPR out of fear of breaking a patient's ribs, or even damaging their professional reputation if wrong. This is called omission bias[5] and must be avoided.

Once the emergency is recognized and the team is mobilized, effective outcomes are the results of deliberate practice. It is not only important to educate the ambulatory center staff about the protocols, but retraining the staff at intervals of six months may be necessary to improve skills and improve retention.[6]

There are several key points which have been shown in recent years to correlate with improved outcomes and should be emphasized in training[1]:

1. Early defibrillation is lifesaving and AED use should not be restricted to trained medical personnel
2. Defibrillation should not be delayed. One rescuer can begin chest compressions while the AED or defibrillator is obtained

3. Incomplete chest recoil is common and full release after each compression should be emphasized
4. "No flow" fraction should be minimized, i.e. continuous CPR maintained
5. Unscheduled mock codes improve mock code performance in hospital personnel
6. Rescuer should be alternated every 2 min to prevent rescuer fatigue which results in deterioration of chest compression quality, specifically depth of compression (>38 mm)
7. It is reasonable to use cognitive aids (checklists) during resuscitation. Caution is advised so that unintentional delay in initiation of the correct protocol does not occur. It is difficult for the event leader to simultaneously lead and read, and thus the role of a reader has been suggested.[7]

In the three drill cases presented, the first patient had a spontaneous non-STEMI related to a primary coronary artery process such as an atherosclerotic plaque rupture, ulceration, fissuring, erosion, or dissection with resulting intraluminal thrombosis. In this case it would be important to make the decision early to transfer the patient to a facility capable of PCI or an in-house transfer to the cardiac catheterization laboratory. The goal of a 90 minute door-to-device time is quite feasible in most cases, since the initial symptoms have been witnessed. However, if this is not practical, then the decision to start fibrinolytic therapy should be considered.

The second patient had STEMI related to stent thrombosis. This presents itself as a sudden dramatic event, and the urgency is even greater to get the patient to a catheterization lab. Stent thrombosis often presents as devastating ventricular arrhythmias and cardiac collapse.

It is important to understand that an estimated 600,000 coronary stents[8] are placed annually in the United States, and that the cumulative incidence of non-cardiac surgery following coronary artery stenting is more than 10% at one year and over 20% at two years.[9] Despite evidence-based guidelines on antiplatelet therapy, there is still much controversy on managing perioperative antiplatelet medication. Even though patients are told by medical staff to stay on their aspirin perioperatively, they often will still discontinue it on their own. The hypercoagulable state induced by the stress of surgery, along with a rebound effect from stopping aspirin, can increase the chances of a late stent thrombosis.[10]

The third case was unstable angina related to ischemic imbalance; the oxygen demand was higher than the supply because of the tachycardia and underlying coronary artery disease and it was unclear whether it would evolve to an MI or not. This patient needs follow-up in a cardiac care unit, and may become unstable at any point.

As anesthesiologists and anesthetists, we are used to taking care of the patients ourselves. It is indeed a paradigm shift to rely on a system to help us take care of these patients, and the key element to saving lives is having systems in place that ensure smooth transfers to the appropriate facilities.

References

1. Hazinski MF, Billi JE, Boettiger BW, Bossaert L, de Caen AR, Deakin CD, Drajer S, Eigel B, Hickey RW, Jacobs I, Kleinman ME, Kloek W, Koster RW, Lim SH, Mancini ME, Montgomery WH, Morley PT, Morrison LJ, Nadkarni VM, O'connor RE, Okada K, Perlman JM, Sayre MR, Shuster M, Soar M, Kjetil S, Travers AH, Wyllie J, Zideman D (2010). Part 1, executive summary: 2010 International Consensus on Cardiopulmonary Resuscitation and Emergency Cardiovascular Care Science with Treatment Recommendations. *Circulation* 122(supp. 2): S250–S275.

2. Fleisher LA, Auerbach AD, Barnason SA, Beckman JA, Bozkurt B, Davila-Roman VG, Gerhard-Herman MD, Holly TA, Kane GC, Marine JE, Nelson MT, Spencer CC, Thompson A, Ting HH, Uretsky BF, Wijeysundera DN (2013). 2014 ACC/AHA guideline on perioperative cardiovascular evaluation and management of patients undergoing noncardiac surgery: a report of the American College of Cardiology/American Heart Association Task Force on Practice Guidelines. *J Am Coll Cardiol* 64(e77–137).

3. Amsterdam EA, Brindis RG, Casey DE Jr, Ganiats TG, Holmes DR Jr, Jaffe AS, Jneid H, Kelly RF, Kontos MC, Levine GN, Liebson PR, Mukherjee D, Peterson ED, Sabatine MS, Smalling RW, Zieman SJ (2014). 2014 ACC/AHA guideline for the management of patients with non–ST-elevation acute coronary syndromes: a report of the American College of Cardiology/American Heart Association Task Force on Practice Guidelines. *Circulation* 64(24): e139–228.

4. O'Gara PT, Ascheim DD, Casey DE Jr, Chung MK, de Lemos JA, Ettinger SM, Fang JC, Fesmire FM, Franklin BA, Granger CB, Krumholz HM, Linderbaum JA, Morrow DA, Newby LK, Ornato JP, Ou N, Radford MJ, Tamis-Holland JE, Tommaso CL, Tracy CM, Woo YJ, Zhao DX (2013). 2013 ACCF/AHA Guideline for the Management of ST-Elevation Myocardial Infarction. *J Am Coll Cardiol* 61: e78–140.

5. Stiegler MP, Tung A (2014). Cognitive Processes in Anesthesiologiy Decision Making. *Anesthesiology* 120 (1): 204–217.

6. Mancini ME, Bhanji F, Billli JE, Dennett J, Finn J, Ma MH, Perkins GD, Rodgers DL, Hazinski MF, Jacobs I, Morley PT (2010). Part 12: education, implementation and teams: 2010 International Consensus on Cardiopulmonary Resuscitation and Emergency Cardiovascular Care Science with Treatment Recommendations. *Circulation* 122 (supp. 2): S539–S581.

7. Goldhaber-Fiebert, SN, Howard, SK. (2013). Implementing Emergency Manuals: Can Cogitive Aids Help Translate Best Practices for Patient Care During Acute Events? *Anesthesia & Analgesia* 117(5): 1149–1161.

8. Epstein AJ, Yang F, Yang L, Groeneveld P (2011). Coronary Revascularization Trends in the United States, 2001–2008. *JAMA* 305(17): 1769–1776.

9. Hawn MT, Richman JR, Itani KM, Plomondon ME, Altom LK, Henderson WG, Bryson CL, Maddox TM (2012). The Incidence and Timing of Noncardiac Surgery after Cardiac Stent Implantation. *Am Coll Surg* 214: 658–667.

10. Lemesle G, Collins S, Waksman R (2010). Drug-Eluting Stents: Issues of Late Stent Thrombosis. *Cardiol Clin* 28: 97–105.

Reversible causes of cardiac arrest

Steven Butz

Introduction

Cardiac arrest can occur for reasons other than ischemic heart disease. The American Heart Association classifies them into the reversible causes of cardiac arrest, the H's and T's. The mnemonic stands for, in this case, hypoxemia, hypovolemia, hydrogen ion (acidosis), hypo-/hyperkalemia, hypothermia, thrombosis (pulmonary and cardiac), toxins, tamponade (cardiac), and tension pneumothorax. A study of European in-hospital cardiac arrest attributed 42% of 258 cardiac arrests to these reversible causes.[1]

This chapter will direct you through scenarios that may be seen in an ambulatory setting that are derived from these etiologies.

Educational objectives

1. Encourage review of situations to identify potentially reversible causes of cardiac arrest.
2. Be able to enumerate causes of reversible arrest.
3. Evaluate clinical setting for presence of diagnostic and therapeutic items to differentiate causes of cardiac arrest.

Scenario 1: Pneumothorax

A 38-year-old male with aggressive testicular cancer presents for central line insertion for chemotherapy. He undergoes an uneventful general anesthetic with propofol, remifentanil, ketorolac, and ondansetron. A laryngeal mask airway is used to control his ventilation.

In the recovery room, the patient gets agitated and is fighting the nursing staff trying to calm him and keep him restrained. The patient screams that he has trouble breathing.

Expected actions:

1. Evaluate monitors for signs of hypoxia and arrhythmias.

2. Apply oxygen.
3. Assess vital signs.

Scenario continued:

The patient is hypotensive with blood pressure 54/28 with heart rate of 138 and oxygen saturation of 82% with 4 l oxygen by facemask.

Expected actions:

1. Assess for jugular venous distension and bilateral breath sounds.
2. Assess EKG waveform for signs of hyperkalemia.
3. Prepare for intubation.
4. Consider bolus of IV fluid.
5. Consider chest x-ray.

Scenario continued:

Suddenly, the patient's eyes roll back into his head and he slumps to the side. ECG rhythm is still sinus tachycardia. There is no pulse.

Expected actions:

1. Call for help.
2. Begin ACLS for pulseless electrical activity (PEA).
3. Assess for cardiac tamponade versus tension pneumothorax during secondary assessment.
4. CPR is to continue to provide perfusion.

Scenario continued:

There are no breath sounds on the left chest, the side with the new central line.

Expected actions:

1. Needle aspiration of air is performed in left chest at second intercostal space anteriorly at the mid-clavicular line.

Perioperative Drill-Based Crisis Management, ed. Steven Butz. Published by Cambridge University Press. © Cambridge University Press 2016.

2. Consider placement of chest tube if available.
3. Ultrasound may be used as a guide for evaluation of pneumothorax.

Scenario continued:

Pulse returns with relief of tension pneumothorax. Plans should be made for transfer to hospital.

Scenario 2: Acidosis and hypovolemia

A 51-year-old, 56 kg female patient with type 1 diabetes has undergone a screening colonoscopy. She successfully completed her prep and had documented her blood sugars at home. Her A-1-c is 7.1, but was running in the 200s in the previous days and not feeling well. After her prep, her glucose was 300–400 mg/dl despite treating with subcutaneous insulin at home. On arrival that morning, her sugar was 275 mg/dl. Your anesthesia colleague was consulted by the gastroenterologist to help get the case completed since the patient wanted it done and had completed her bowel preparation. The anesthesiologist agreed to do the case since the 275 mg/dl reading was improved from the previous day. Propofol sedation was given and a bolus of 1 l of lactated Ringer's solution was given prior to starting.

Your colleague left due to a family emergency and you are called to the recovery room 30 min after the patient arrived. She has not woken up.

Expected actions:

1. Assess the patient and review history.
2. Check blood glucose.
3. Check ketones if available. May require placing urinary catheter to check urine dipstick.
4. Assess for hypovolemia and give bolus of normal saline.

Scenario continued:

Glucose is "high" on glucometer. Before patient can be aroused, the EKG shows peaked T-waves that evolve into pulseless ventricular tachycardia.

Expected actions:

1. Call for help.
2. Begin CPR and ACLS protocol for pulseless VT/VF. *CPR needs to be continued throughout administration of medications until pulse is restored.*
3. Advanced airway management. Intubation is indicated for patients undergoing CPR; *alternative methods of oxygenation may be used if personnel with intubation skills are unavailable.*
4. Perform secondary assessment after initial treatment with focus on treatment of acidosis from diabetic ketoacidosis (DKA) and hypovolemia.

Scenario continued:

Shocks have been unsuccessful. A colleague recommends placing a Foley catheter and gets dark urine with positive ketones on a dipstick test. No triggering agents were used. Your colleague also recommends hanging hetastarch since she is obviously dry and to give a 15 unit bolus of IV insulin.

Expected actions:

1. Continue CPR and ACLS.
2. Begin treatment for hyperkalemia.
   a. calcium
   b. regular insulin IV
3. Give fluid bolus of 1 l of normal saline.

Scenario continued:

Next round of shocks restore normal sinus rhythm. Patient is still ventilated. There has been no urine production.

Expected actions:

1. Make arrangements for transfer.
2. Blood gas may be drawn if possible to process.
3. Continue volume resuscitation with normal saline.
4. May begin insulin treatment with either normal saline drip at 0.05 units/kg/h or ultra rapid insulin 0.5 units /kg subcutaneous injection.

Scenario continued:

The drill would end when ambulance arrives. Facility personnel likely to go along to provide report and ventilation.

Scenario 3: Anaphylaxis

A 17-year-old female is undergoing a left ACL repair. She has a known egg allergy and a history of asthma and psoriasis. A femoral nerve catheter was placed preoperatively and the procedure is being performed under general anesthesia. The anesthetic used is a total IV anesthetic (TIVA) due to history of severe PONV with previous surgery. She is being maintained on propofol and ketamine infusions with nitrous oxide, ketorolac, dexamethasone, and ondansetron. A dose of cefazolin was administered preoperatively. The airway is managed with a supraglottic airway.

Approximately 15 min into the procedure, the oxygen saturation has dropped to 91% and tidal volumes are decreased to 200 ml.

Expected actions:

1. Examine the patient by auscultating the lungs and looking at the skin for rashes.
2. Look at the end-tidal CO_2 tracing for evidence of bronchospasm.
3. Hand-ventilate and administer albuterol for bronchospasm.

Scenario continued:

Blood pressure cycles and is now 48/23. Heart rate is 118 bpm.

Expected actions:

1. Epinephrine 100–200 mcg IV administered.
2. Volume expansion with crystalloid.
3. Review of possible allergic triggers: propofol (egg allergy), ketorolac (asthma-related aspirin allergy), antibiotic, latex.
4. Work to remove possible trigger.

Scenario continued:

Patient's cardiac rhythm deteriorates into ventricular fibrillation. Patient's face is noticeably edematous.

Expected actions:

1. Begin ACLS protocol for VT/VF.
2. Proceed with cardiac compression and intubation.
3. Administer high-dose epinephrine.
4. Surgery should be closed/aborted.

Scenario continued:

Sinus rhythm returns after 2 cycles of epinephrine and shocks. Patient remains hypotensive.

Expected actions:

1. Epinephrine drip should be started.
2. Patient should be dosed with higher-dose dexamethasone. Consider adding diphenhydramine and H_2 blocker.

Scenario continued:

The drill ends with arrangements for transfer and completion of secondary survey.

Debriefing

1. Identify up to three or more things the team felt went well with the scenario.
2. Identify up to three or more things the team felt they should have done differently.
3. What equipment was difficult to locate or use?
4. Were the H's and T's addressed early?
5. Were suggestions from staff taken and considered?
6. What aspects of patient history or case scenario were there to lead to correct diagnosis?
7. What processes worked well and what needs to be improved?

Discussion

Although the protocols for resuscitation for ventricular fibrillation/tachycardia and pulseless electrical activity continue regardless of cause, identifying the etiology may lead to a successful resolution more quickly. The cause of cardiac arrest in hospital is most often primary cardiac disease, but the H's and T's account for 42% of arrests.[1] The numbers are likely to be different in the outpatient setting and actually may be higher for non-cardiac causes as patients with severe cardiac disease are selected away from an ambulatory setting. Aspects of the H's and T's relevant to the scenarios presented will be described below.

Scenario 1: Pneumothorax

Hypoxemia by itself may lead to cardiac arrest. The etiology probably combines other components of the H's and T's. As a person is deprived of oxygen, anaerobic metabolism will begin. This contributes to acidosis. The high oxygen consumption of the heart makes it particularly vulnerable to low oxygen levels. If the cause is combined with poor ventilation, the hypercarbia will further increase acidosis making the myocardium more vulnerable to arrhythmias. Shifts in pH will also affect potassium levels, causing more irritability. Toxins can cause hypoxemia as in the case of cyanide or carbon monoxide.

Treatment of hypoxia is reversing the primary cause. For ambulatory surgery, the most likely successful maneuver will be re-establishing a patent airway. This may be more difficult in a patient with a history of obstructive sleep apnea as they are at higher risk for desaturation in the recovery room than the healthy patient. Toxins each have an individual treatment, and identification of the toxin will go a long way to determine the next steps in treatment.

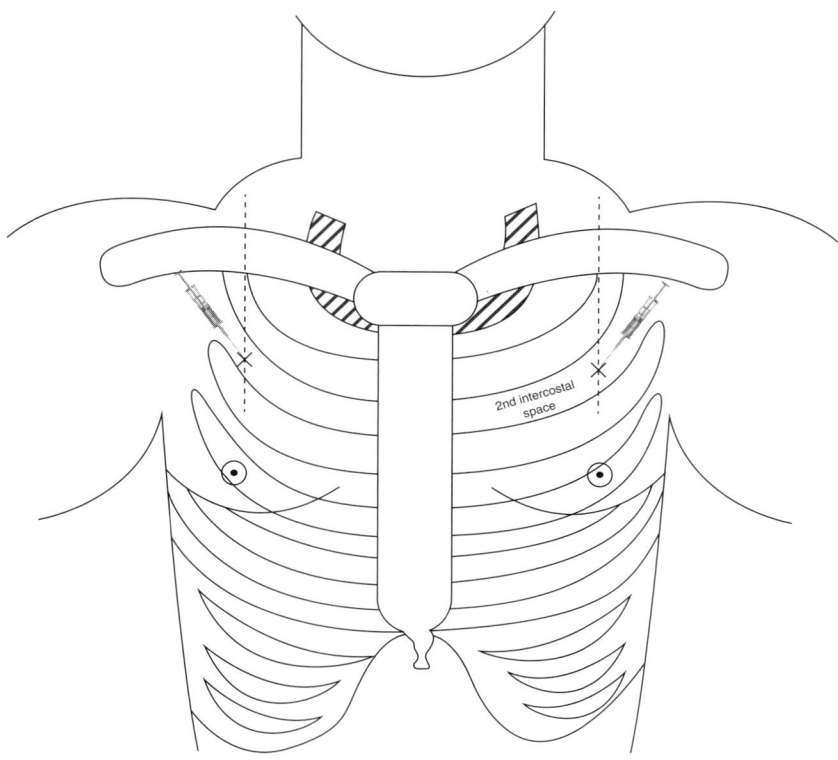

Figure 2.1 Approach used to place a needle to relieve a tension pneumothorax

In our case, the hypoxemia was most likely due to either a tension pneumothorax or even a pericardial effusion. Either can present as an acute or chronic problem, each with different treatments. For this patient, the onset was acute and needed emergent treatment. On physical exam, tracheal deviation away from the affected side is seen. Jugular venous distension and hyperresonance to percussion are late findings.[2] The diagnosis can be difficult in an ambulatory setting. A chest film can be performed during a code to diagnose a pneumothorax. However, a skilled ultrasonographer may also be able to diagnose it with an ultrasound machine.[3] An article comparing AP chest films with non-radiologist sonographers demonstrated equivalent sensitivity and specificity. A tension pneumothorax may be diagnosed by ultrasound when there is an absence of lung sliding and B lines are present. B lines are seen in an anteriomedial view in the mid-clavicular line. These are vertical lines that arise from the pleural line and extend to the lower edge of the screen.[4]

Treatment of a tension pneumothorax is with a 14- or 16-gauge needle inserted into the second intercostal space in the mid-clavicular line. This will release the pressure with a rush.[2] After relief, there needs to be careful monitoring to ensure that there is no recurrence of

the flap-valve mechanism causing the initial pneumothorax, requiring a chest tube placement.

A cardiac tamponade would be possible if there were proximal rupture of the vasculature or atrium with the wire used to place the central line. Hemodynamically significant tamponade may show the signs of jugular venous distension (JVD) and pulsus paradoxus. The JVD reflects the higher right atrial filling pressures. Pulsus paradoxus is an exaggeration of the decrease in blood pressure that occurs with respiration. Typically, blood pressure drops 10 mmHg when increased negative intra-thoracic pressure decreases the left atrial filling. With tamponade, filling is further restricted and the blood pressure drop is more pronounced.[5] Other signs of tamponade are dyspnea, tachycardia, and decreased heart tones. Diagnosis with ultrasound is made when effusion is identified and there is collapse of the right chamber size in the cardiac cycle. These findings are very accurate for the diagnosis.[3]

Treatment for cardiac tamponade should include airway management and CPR as needed. The patient should be placed with chest elevated 45°. The perixyphoid area should be prepped and draped. Ideally, a 16- or 18-gauge cardiac needle about 15 cm long should be attached via a stopcock to a 50 ml syringe.

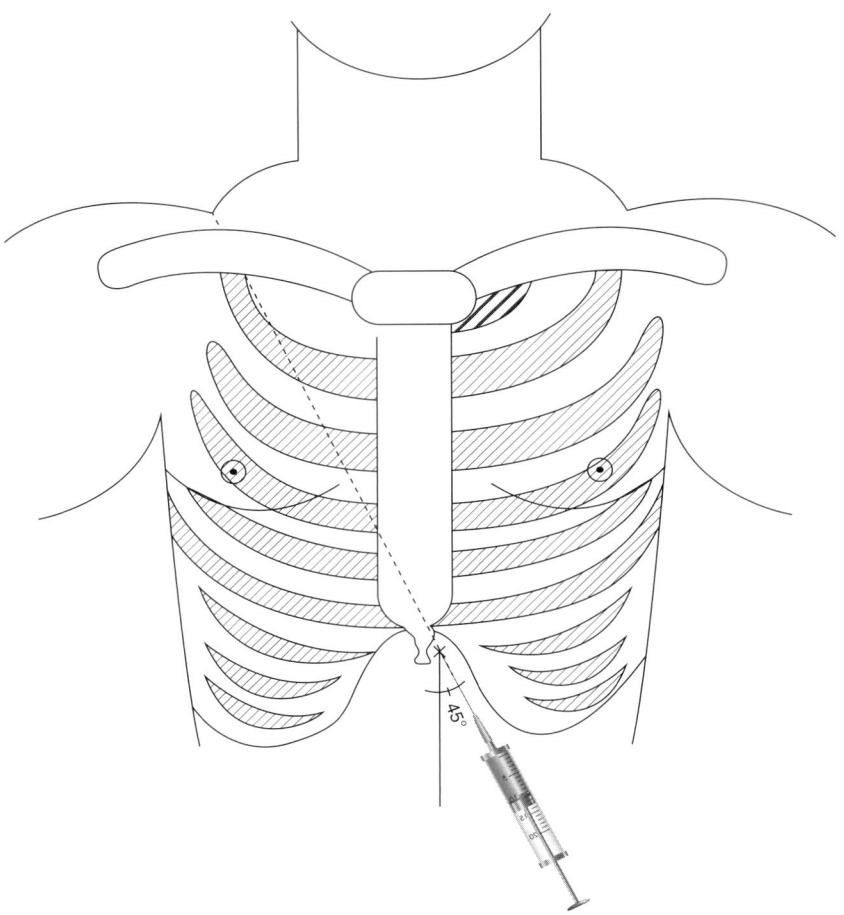

Figure 2.2 Approach used to aspirate fluid causing cardiac tamponade

Using ultrasound or careful EKG monitoring, the needle is advanced from just inferior-lateral to the left of the xyphoid at a 45° angle toward the left mid-clavicle. Once the pericardium is entered (it may be felt by the person advancing the needle), blood is withdrawn. Symptoms may reverse quickly even after a small amount of blood is withdrawn. A clamp may be used to stabilize the needle at the skin or a catheter may be threaded in to withdraw the blood. The EKG should be viewed looking for evidence of entry into the ventricle or atrium. Ventricular penetration will cause ST elevations and atrial penetration may cause PR elevation.[2]

Scenario 2: Acidosis and hypovolemia

The issues woven into this scenario include hypovolemia, acidosis, diabetes, and coverage issues. The resulting controversies are the care for ketoacidosis and fluid resuscitation. Recognition of hyperkalemia would be critical to success, as would the correct treatment.

Hypovolemia in an ambulatory surgery center may be present for many different reasons. Fasting patients are already dry, but a healthy patient should be able to compensate. Patients on diuretics or having bowel preparations will be further depleted. Relative hypovolemia may occur in cases of vasodilation caused by sympathetic blockade or anaphylaxis and shock. Life-threatening hypovolemia in the surgical setting can be from extreme or unnoticed blood loss. Bleeding from a laparoscopic procedure may continue until the patient decompensates.

Volume replacement is the first treatment until the cause of hypovolemia is addressed. The fluid of choice is controversial when considering crystalloid versus colloid. Previous thought was that only one third of administered crystalloids stayed intravascular. Newer data suggest that more like 70% remains intravascular. This fact, combined with studies of the endothelial glycocalyx, demonstrates that inflammation makes it more permeable than was believed.[6] Recent work comparing colloids and crystalloids in trauma demonstrates either no significant improvement in morbidity or mortality with colloids, but there is a delayed increase in mortality with colloids and traumatic brain injury patients. Two large studies, SAFE and ALBIOS, supported albumin for resuscitation of ICU patients with septic shock.

Hydroxyethyl starches are one of the more commonly available colloids for ambulatory centers due to availability and easy storage. Earlier starch solutions were associated with renal dysfunction, pruritus, hyperbilirubinemia, and coagulopathy. Reformulated solutions with lower oncotic pressures and smaller molecular weight starches improved their safety. However, high-dose starch resuscitation remains expensive and has associated nephrotoxicity.

Crystalloids are not entirely benign. Recent research has implicated poor outcomes associated with hyperchloremia when normal saline solutions are used. Even balanced salt solutions are not free of negative characteristics. Frequently, organic anions are substituted for chlorine and bicarbonate ions. These can lead to metabolic alkalosis and hypertonicity.

Overall, the best immediate resuscitation is with available crystalloids according to Advanced Trauma Life Support.[7] Lactated Ringer's would be better than normal saline. Decompensated blood losses are best replaced with blood products, but these are typically not readily available at an ambulatory facility. Even these cases benefit from crystalloid to restore perfusion until blood can be administered.[6]

Diabetic ketoacidosis (DKA) can occur at relatively low blood sugars in a type 1 diabetes patient. It may occur in type 2, but usually in more extreme blood sugar ranges. Risks for DKA include illness (this patient had a viral syndrome preoperatively), dehydration, lack of or underdose of insulin for given carbohydrate intake, stress, and steroids. After suspicion, diagnosis would include a high glucose and acidosis. Since not many ambulatory centers have a laboratory to run blood gases, presence of ketones by urine dipstick can substitute. However, just dehydration (from bowel preparations) can precipitate ketosis, but not necessarily DKA. Mental status changes may indicate more severe DKA.

Treatment of DKA is best undertaken in a hospital setting with complete laboratory services available.

Once DKA is identified, volume resuscitation with normal saline is started. Estimates are that adult patients in DKA are down 6–9 l of fluid. Insulin is not given until hydration has started and potassium is at least 3.3 mmol/l. If potassium is less than 3.3 mmol/l, potassium replacement is continued until levels are above 3.3. This step alone prevents treatment at an ambulatory center without ability to measure potassium. ECG changes may indicate high potassium levels, but are not diagnostic. IV solutions are changed to 5% dextrose 0.45 NS and are run in tandem with insulin infusions once glucose is under 250 mg/dl. Treatment is converted to subcutaneous insulin and oral hydration/nutrition when bicarbonate levels normalize and anion gap is 10–12.[8] In the ASC setting, the first steps of reaching a diagnosis, hydrating and stabilizing, are the goals while arranging for transport to a hospital setting.

Scenario 3: Anaphylaxis

Anaphylaxis can carry a mortality rate of up to 9%. The presentation can be varied, but may include rash, angioedema, tachycardia, hypotension, and bronchospasm. The incidence ranges from 0.5 to 2.9 per 10,000 patients. The operating room also is a point where many drugs from different classes are given very close together. There can also be intimate exposure to drugs via irrigation solutions and latex. These factors can make identifying the offending agent very difficult.

There are allergic and non-allergic causes of anaphylaxis. The allergic mechanisms are mediated via the immune system by IgE (or IgG or immunoglobin/complement reaction). The non-allergic type may be direct activation of the complement system, direct action on mast cells causing degranulation, or dysfunction of arachidonic acid metabolism. Under anesthesia, 66% of anaphylaxis reactions are immunologically derived. Either mechanism is treated with epinephrine and the more quickly it is given, the better the patient outcome will be.

Patients with a latex allergy or signs/symptoms of latex allergies are at higher risk for anaphylaxis. This includes allergies to associated foods such as kiwi, avocado, banana, pineapple, chestnut, passion fruit, or buckwheat. Asthmatics with nasal polyps have an increased chance of aspirin or NSAID allergy. And patients with an atypic history (psoriasis or eczema) may have an increased risk of allergic reactions. Systemic mastocytosis sufferers can have anaphyloid reactions that are not mediated by the immune system.

These are treated with epinephrine, too, and patients may be on steroids for disease management.

The drugs most likely to cause a reaction are neuromuscular blocking agents and antibiotics. Queries for reactions to these agents should be sought preoperatively. Propofol uses the lecithin component of eggs in its production, so an egg protein allergy does not prevent the use of propofol as an anesthetic agent.

Once suspected, anaphylaxis is treated by first removing the triggering agent if it is known. Depending on the severity of the anaphylaxis, diphenhydramine or epinephrine is given. Skin-only manifestations can be treated with diphenhydramine 0.5–1 mg/kg IV. More severe symptoms are treated with epinephrine. Lower-grade doses are 10–20 mcg IV in adults. More severe symptoms can be treated with 100–200 mcg IV. Doses can be repeated until symptoms begin to resolve. Volume expansion with crystalloid should be used to treat vasodilation and hypotension. Bronchospasm is treated with beta-agonists such as albuterol (inhaled) or epinephrine (IV). Steroids can be given, but are not useful in the immediate resuscitation period. They will help prevent late-phase shock and bronchospasm. Most cardiovascular collapse is due to asphyxiation from airway edema. Intubation should occur early in the treatment course to secure the airway.

Tryptase levels can be drawn to confirm an allergic cause for the anaphylaxis. Skin testing or serum testing should not be done for several weeks following to get a clearer picture of the causative agent if one is not already suspected.[9]

References

1. E Sinz and K Navarro (Eds.) *Advanced Cardiovascular Life Support Provider Manual.* American Heart Association. May 2011.
2. GR Braen (Ed.). *Manual of Emergency Medicine Sixth Edition.* Lippincott Williams & Wilkins. Philadelphia, PA. 2011.
3. W Ding, Y Shen, J Yang, X He, M Zhang. Diagnosis of pneumothorax by radiography and ultrasound. *Chest* (2011) 40; 859–866.
4. Giovanni Volpicelli. Usefulness of emergency ultrasound in nontraumatic cardiac arrest. *American Journal of Emergency Medicine* (2011) 29; 216–223.
5. E Argulian, F Messerti. Misconception and facts about pericardial effusion and tamponade. *The American Journal of Medicine* (2013) 126; 858–861.
6. JA Myburgh. Fluid resuscitation in acute medicine: what is the current situation? *Journal of Internal Medicine* (2015) 277; 58–68.
7. I Kwan, F Bunn, P Chinnock, I Roberts. Timing and volume of fluid administration for patients with bleeding (review). *The Cochrane Collaboration* (2014); 1–18.
8. AR Gosmanov, EO Gosmanova, E Dillard-Cannon. Management of adult diabetic ketoacidosis. *Diabetes, Metabolic Syndrome and Obesity; Targets and Therapy* (2014) 7: 255–264.
9. V Regnier Galvao, P Giavina-Bianchi, M Castells. Perioperative anaphylaxis. *Curr Allergy Asthma Rep* (2014) 14; 452.

Malignant hyperthermia

Fatima Ahmad

Introduction

Malignant hyperthermia (MH) is a rare but fulminant reaction to inhalational anesthetics and succinylcholine, and in some instances to heat stroke and exercise. It is a medical emergency that can be fatal if a coordinated team response to treat it is not initiated in timely fashion. Every ambulatory surgery center should have its own MH crisis response plan tailored to its specific needs. This plan should be practiced during periodic simulations and MH drills.

MH symptoms can occur during or after surgery. In addition to the operating room, MH can present in the recovery room, intensive care unit, emergency room, or dental and surgical offices.

Four scenarios are presented here to help understand and prepare for the rapid diagnosis and management of MH in different situations.

Educational objectives

1. Ensure the prevention of occurrence of MH in patients with known susceptibility to MH
2. Early recognition of MH
3. Prompt and effective management of MH

Scenario 1: Adult case in freestanding center

An 18-year-old female presents in a freestanding ambulatory surgery center for cosmetic breast surgery to correct significant breast asymmetry. She has no significant past medical history and has never had general anesthesia in the past. There is no family history of any anesthesia-related complications. She is not on any medications and does not have any known allergies. She weighs 65 kg.

The anesthetic plan is general anesthesia with laryngeal mask airway (LMA). She is premedicated with midazolam 2 mg IV, standard ASA monitors are placed, and induction is performed with 200 mg propofol and 5 ml 1% lidocaine IV (to blunt the pain associated with propofol). LMA is placed uneventfully. End-tidal carbon dioxide ($ETCO_2$) is confirmed and manual ventilation is initiated until return of spontaneous ventilation. Sevoflurane with a mixture of oxygen and air is used for maintenance of anesthesia. A nasal temperature probe is placed and the temperature is noted to be 36.8°C.

After resumption of spontaneous ventilation, it is noted that tidal volumes are inadequate; $ETCO_2$ is 55 and oxygen saturation is 94% with a heart rate of 85–90/min. Manual ventilation is found to be difficult at this time and laryngospasm is diagnosed. LMA is removed and manual ventilation with 100% oxygen and positive pressure is attempted. Oxygen saturation decreases to 88%. Patient is still difficult to ventilate. Succinylcholine (70 mg) is administered and the patient is intubated. End-tidal CO_2 and bilateral breath sounds are confirmed. Mechanical ventilation is started with a rate of 16 and tidal volume of 600; sevoflurane is resumed. Oxygen saturation improves to 94%. Patient's heart rate and $ETCO_2$ continue to rise and peak airway pressure is noted to be 38 cm H_2O. Respiratory rate and tidal volumes are both increased.

Vital signs at this time are noted to be:

1. HR 110/min
2. BP 110/70
3. O_2 saturation 95%
4. $ETCO_2$ 75
5. Temperature 38°C
6. On palpation of masseter muscle, rigidity is felt.

Perioperative Drill-Based Crisis Management, ed. Steven Butz. Published by Cambridge University Press. © Cambridge University Press 2016.

Expected actions:

1. Discontinue inhalational anesthetic agent
2. Start hyperventilation with 100% oxygen at high flow rate
3. Initiate MH response plan by informing the surgical team and calling for help
4. MH cart and crash cart should both be brought to OR
5. Assign tasks to everyone
6. Start mixing dantrolene
7. Start cooling of patient.

Scenario continued:

After help has arrived, it is noted on the monitor that temperature has increased to 39°C, blood pressure is 70/40, and rhythm has deteriorated to ventricular tachycardia.

Expected actions:

1. Check pulse
2. Give 2.5 mg/kg IV dantrolene
3. Start another IV if enough personnel are available
4. Treat hyperthermia by placing ice packs in groin and axilla and administering IV cold saline.

Scenario continued:

There is no pulse.

Expected actions:

1. Initiate pulseless ventricular tachycardia treatment as per ACLS protocol. Continue CPR until return of pulse. Administer ACLS medications as indicated
2. Continue MH protocol during ACLS
   – Administration of dantrolene.
   – Cooling the patient.
3. If no blood gas testing capabilities are available, start treatment for hyperkalemia and acidosis empirically.
4. 24 h MH hotline (800-644-9737) should be called by a designated person
5. 9-1-1 should be called and a clear, detailed message should be delivered by a designated person
6. Family should be informed about the situation by a person specifically designated for this purpose.

Scenario continued:

There is return of pulse with restoration of sinus rhythm. Vital signs at this time are:

1. HR 130 per min
2. BP 90/50 mmHg
3. $ETCO_2$ 90
4. Oxygen saturation 94%
5. Temp 40°C.

Expected actions:

1. Give another dose of dantrolene
2. Continue hyperventilation
3. Start arterial line if available
4. Continue cooling methods including placement of nasogastric tube and gastric lavage with cold saline, placement of ice packs over various body parts, and IV administration of cold saline
5. Urinary catheter should be placed
6. If patient is being taken to Post Anesthesia Care Unit (PACU), the nurses should be well prepared to handle MH management
7. Transfer arrangements with the receiving hospital should be made informing them of the patient's condition, and need for ICU bed and mechanical ventilation.

Scenario continued:

Drill ends when two doses of dantrolene 2.5 mg/kg are administered, temperature comes down to 38°C, and $ETCO_2$ is improving.

Scenario 2: Adult case in freestanding center

At a freestanding surgery center, in the PACU you are taking care of a 48-year-old, 70 kg patient who has had inguinal hernia repair under general anesthesia. You were told in the postoperative report that he does not have any significant past medical history, no known drug allergies and had an uneventful anesthetic course during which he was given propofol, fentanyl, oxygen/nitrous oxide, and sevoflurane.

On arrival to PACU his vital signs are:

1. HR 88 per min
2. BP 118/85
3. Resp 18 per min
4. Temp 37.1°C
5. Oxygen saturation 98% on room air
6. He complains of pain with a visual analog scale (VAS) 6/10.

Fentanyl (50 mcg) is administered with improvement in VAS to 4/10. However, because his heart rate and blood pressure are climbing up and 10 min after the first dose of fentanyl, you administer a second dose of 50 mcg. He reports pain relief of 0–1/10 at this time. Approximately 30 min after his arrival to PACU, he complains of shortness of breath, palpitations, and feeling uncomfortably warm; his face is flushed and his lips appeared cyanosed. Vital signs at this time are as follows:

- HR 130/min
- BP 140/90
- Resp 30/min
- Temp 39°C
- Oxygen saturation 94% on room air.

Expected actions:

1. Assess patient for causes of decreased perfusion, hypoxia, fever
2. Develop differential diagnosis.

Scenario continued:

Patient becomes unresponsive. His heart rate is 140 and blood pressure 100/55.

Expected actions:

1. Start mask ventilation with bag until intubated
2. Make sure that a non-depolarizing muscle relaxant is available to facilitate intubation
3. Intubate and confirm $ETCO_2$ with end-tidal monitor
4. Continue manual ventilation.

Scenario continued:

$ETCO_2$ reading on monitor is 73–78 mmHg. Patient is becoming rigid.

Expected actions:

1. Initiate MH response plan by calling for help and informing the anesthesiologist
2. Remove patient's blankets immediately
3. MH cart and crash cart should both be brought in
4. Assign tasks to everyone
5. Start preparation of dantrolene
6. Start cooling of the patient
7. Start dantrolene administration (2.5 mg/kg initial dose)
8. Someone should prepare an anesthesia machine for mechanical ventilation if available. Put on a new anesthesia breathing circuit and CO_2 absorbent and remove vaporizers of inhalational agents
9. Bring the anesthesia machine to PACU from the operating room or take the patient to operating room (whichever is quicker and easier) so mechanical ventilation can be started.

Scenario continued:

As the endotracheal tube is connected to the anesthesia circuit, it is noted that the $ETCO_2$ is 90. Peak airway pressures is 40 cmH$_2$O. Skin appears mottled. EKG shows frequent PVCs. Temperature is 40°C, HR 144, blood pressure 95/50, and oxygen saturation 95% on FiO$_2$ of 100%.

Expected actions:

1. Start hyperventilation
2. Continue to administer dantrolene
3. Continue cooling methods
4. Start another IV
5. Start arterial line if available
6. Draw arterial blood samples to test blood gas if available (consider drawing if transferring)
7. If no blood gas testing capability is available, empirically treat metabolic acidosis and hyperkalemia
8. 24 hour MH hotline (800-644-9737) should be called by a designated person
9. 911 should be called and a clear detailed message should be delivered by a designated person
10. Family should be updated about the situation by a designated person.

Scenario continued:

Drill ends when $ETCO_2$ starts to come down and temperature is decreased to 38°C.

Scenario 3: Pediatric case in endoscopy center

A 14-year-old male, 62 kg, is undergoing an endoscopy for celiac disease. He desires a general anesthetic so he had a mask induction with sevoflurane and was converted to IV propofol for maintenance after the IV was placed. There are no known allergies or previous anesthetics. He is spontaneously breathing with nasal cannula oxygen at 4 l/min. When the endoscopist attempts to place the endoscope, she is unable to open the patient's mouth. A 0.5 mcg/kg bolus of fentanyl was given just prior to insertion attempt. Vital signs have been stable.

Expected actions:

1. Assess for depth of anesthesia
2. Assess for rigidity in skeletal muscles
3. Differential is masseter spasm versus narcotic-induced rigidity versus light anesthesia.

Scenario continued:

A bolus of propofol does not relieve the jaw spasm. Mask ventilation is easy via the anesthesia circuit as the patient went apneic with the bolus. Ventricular ectopy has begun.

Expected actions:

1. Call for code cart, malignant hyperthermia cart, and additional help
2. Consider abandoning procedure
3. Confirm triggering agents have been stopped.

Scenario continued:

Before patient can recover from propofol sedation, ventricular fibrillation occurs. The mouth is still clamped tightly shut.

Expected actions:

1. Begin ACLS protocols for ventricular fibrillation and CPR
2. Anticipate intubation if jaw slackens from loss of perfusion
3. Do NOT give succinylcholine
4. Dantrolene should be mixed for administration at 5 mg/kg IV
5. Defibrillation should be performed.

Scenario continued:

The jaw is still tight despite giving an intubating dose of rocuronium. The patient is still in ventricular fibrillation after two shocks. $ETCO_2$ is variable, but present.

Expected actions:

1. Rescue breathing via bag/mask should be maintained
2. Fibrillation algorithm should be continued

3. Dantrolene should be administered until jaw relaxes. Rocuronium only works on neuromuscular junction and masseter spasm is due to myopathic process
4. CPR should continue
5. Active cooling measures should be performed
6. A urinary catheter should be placed.

Scenario continued:

The urine is tea-colored and the fibrillation converted to sinus tachycardia after fourth shock. Intubation was successful after jaw relaxed. $ETCO_2$ per the anesthesia monitor is 72 mmHg. There is a palpable pulse and blood pressure is 94/51.

Expected actions:

1. Hospital transfer and ambulance should be arranged
2. Anesthesia personnel should accompany patient on transfer
3. Monitor urine output to prevent kidney damage
4. Start hyperventilation
5. Continue to administer dantrolene
6. Continue cooling methods
7. Start another IV
8. Start arterial line if available
9. Draw arterial blood samples to test blood gas if available (consider drawing if transferring)
10. If no blood gas testing capability is available, empirically treat metabolic acidosis and hyperkalemia
11. 24 h MH hotline (800-644-9737) should be called by a designated person
12. Family should be updated about the situation by a designated person.

Scenario 4: Adult in freestanding surgery center

A 32-year-old, 85 kg man is scheduled to have right arthroscopic ACL repair in a freestanding surgery center. His past medical history is significant for severe gastrointestinal reflux disease (GERD). He has had general anesthesia for tonsillectomy when he was 7 years old without any complications. There is no family history of anesthesia-related problems. He takes omeprazole once a day and there are no known drug allergies.

Options for anesthesia are discussed with him. Patient prefers general anesthesia. Uneventful femoral nerve block is performed with 30 ml of 0.5% bupivacaine with 1:200,000 epinephrine before induction of anesthesia. He is premedicated with midazolam 2 mg IV, and standard ASA monitors are placed. Rapid-sequence induction is performed with propofol 200 mg, fentanyl 150 mcg, and 160 mg succinylcholine. He is easily intubated, with immediate confirmation of $ETCO_2$ with bilateral breath sounds. Mechanical ventilation is started at a rate of 12 breaths/min and tidal volume of 700 ml. Anesthesia is maintained on desflurane with a 1:1 mixture of oxygen and nitrous oxide. Antibiotic is administered. An upper body warming blanket is turned on and the surgeon starts positioning the knee. He comments that probably the patient is not adequately anesthetized, as both knees feel stiff.

Expected actions:

1. Depth of anesthesia is assessed
2. Consider increasing anesthesia or giving muscle relaxant
3. Consider muscle rigidity from other sources such as narcotic or abnormal response to succinylcholine
4. Malignant hyperthermia should be mentioned, but perhaps not acted on.

Scenario continued:

General anesthesia is deepened by increasing the desflurane concentration and a non-depolarizing muscle relaxant is also administered to improve relaxation. It is noted at this time that the heart rate has increased to 110/min – it was 90/min just after induction. Fentanyl 100 mg is given. Heart rate continues to increase and now the $ETCO_2$ is also climbing up from 40 mmHg immediately after induction to 70 mmHg. Temperature is 36.9°C. Surgeon complains again about the stiffness of the knees. An increase in peak airway pressures from 25 to 35 is noticed. MH is suspected and on palpation, the jaw is found to be very stiff. Diagnosis of MH is made.

Vital signs at this time are:

– HR 120/min
– BP 130/90
– O_2 saturation 98%
– $ETCO_2$ 75
– Temperature 37.8°C.

Expected actions:

1. Discontinue inhalational anesthetic agent
2. Start hyperventilation with 100% oxygen at high flow rate
3. Initiate MH response plan by informing the surgical team and calling for help
4. MH cart and crash cart should both be brought to OR
5. Assign tasks to everyone
6. Start mixing dantrolene
7. Remove warming blanket and start cooling of patient.

Scenario continued:

After help has arrived, it is noted that temperature has increased to 38.5°C and $ETCO_2$ is increased to 80. Blood pressure is 140/100.

Expected actions:

1. Give first dose of dantrolene at 2.5 mg/kg I/V
2. Treat hyperthermia by placing ice packs in groin and axilla and place orogastric/nasogastric tube for cold lavage.

Scenario continued:

IV site is found to be infiltrated as first dose of dantrolene was being given.

Expected actions:

1. Immediately look for another suitable vein and start IV line again
2. Give 2.5 mg/kg dantrolene full dose
3. Continue MH protocol including cooling off the patient
4. MH hotline should be called by a designated person
5. Emergency Medical Services (EMS) should be called and a clear, detailed message should be delivered by a designated person
6. Family should be informed about the situation by a person specifically designated for this purpose.

Scenario continued:

Patient starts to cough and buck and vital signs are as follows:

- HR 100/min
- BP 130/60
- O_2 saturation 98% in room air
- $ETCO_2$ 60
- Temperature 37.4°C.

Expected actions:

1. Stop cooling measures
2. Start IV sedation
3. Continue hyperventilation
4. Foley catheter should be placed
5. If patient is being taken to PACU, the nurses should be well prepared to handle MH management
6. Transfer arrangements with the receiving hospital should be made informing them of the patient's condition, and need for ICU bed and mechanical ventilation.

Scenario continued:

Drill ends as temperature and $ETCO_2$ are improving.

Debriefing

1. Identify up to three or more things the team felt went well with the scenario.
2. Identify up to three or more things the team felt they should have done differently.
3. What emergency supplies were difficult to locate or use?
4. Were dantrolene and its diluent stocked together and easily accessible in the MH cart?
5. Could staff find three bags of cold saline easily or they had to use room temperature saline?
6. How long did it take to administer first dose of dantrolene from the time MH was diagnosed?
7. How long did it take to place ice packs on patient's body from the time MH was diagnosed?
8. Were the receiving hospital and family informed in a timely manner?
9. What was missing, that the facility would need, to fully care for the patient?
10. If presented with a similar case, what would the staff do differently next time?

Convey the lessons learned from these scenarios and generalize them so they can apply the lesson to other, real-life situations.

Discussion

The most important thing for managing any emergent situation is its anticipation and preparedness ahead of time. Not only should there be a plan to anesthetize a known MH-susceptible patient, but all members of the surgery center should also be well trained and prepared to handle an MH crisis. There should be an existing arrangement with a nearby hospital regarding a transfer plan. There have been instances when patients developed MH during surgery in ambulatory setup and later died in the hospital. This could have happened due to inability to continue treatment and adequate monitoring during the process of transferring to the hospital. According to a study done by Rosero et al, there are about 500–600 MH cases per year in the United States, and mortality from MH is about 5% where the patient was admitted for routine elective surgery.[2] In comparison with this, the mortality is 20% for patients who are transferred to the hospital from ambulatory surgery centers or other hospitals.

The Malignant Hyperthermia Association of the United States (MHAUS) has established definitive protocols for treating MH and these are considered the standard of care for treatment. The information about the recognition and treatment of an MH crisis in a freestanding surgery center and while moving the patient to a hospital is taken directly from the MHAUS guidelines.[3]

What is malignant hyperthermia?

Denborough first described malignant hyperthermia in 1962 when he reported recurrent deaths in the members of a family after exposure to anesthesia. Since then, much has been written in the literature about MH. Malignant hyperthermia is the expression of a genetic variation in some individuals, which gives rise to a life-threatening hypermetabolic response to some drugs used in anesthesia. These drugs are also called triggers and include the potent inhalational anesthetics and succinylcholine. Malignant hyperthermia is an autosomal dominant disease, which means that the siblings and offspring of a patient with MH susceptibility usually have a 50% chance of inheriting a defective gene and they can be susceptible to MH.

MH susceptibility (MHS) is conferred by specific inherited mutations, most commonly related to the ryanodine receptor (type 1) gene.[4] Ryanodine receptor (RYR1) is located on the sarcoplasmic reticulum of the skeletal muscle and calcium is stored here. Opening of RYR1 results in increased intracellular calcium levels and muscle contractions. Opening of RYR1 is mediated by L-type calcium channels in response to increases in intracellular calcium levels. There are two RYR sites associated with changing calcium concentrations. The A-site (high-affinity calcium-binding site) mediates RYR opening while the I-site (lower-affinity site) mediates its closing. Magnesium affects the closing of RYR1 by its affinity for both A- and I-sites. When there is a mutation in RYR1, there is a drastic increase in calcium affinity at the A-site and a decrease in magnesium affinity in response to MH triggering agents. This results in greatly increased calcium release in the muscle cell and sustained muscle contraction. The reabsorption of this calcium requires large amounts of ATP, resulting in generation of excessive heat and cellular hypoxia. ATP depletion and high temperature damage muscle cells (rhabdomyolysis), resulting in leakage of potassium, myoglobin, creatine kinase, creatine, and phosphate into the circulation. Other mutations resulting in the same processes have also been described.[5]

Clinical presentation

The pathophysiologic process described above results in a hypermetabolic response when a susceptible individual is exposed to triggering agents. *This response is characterized by an unexplained increase in end-tidal carbon dioxide concentration among other early warning signs.*

Early warning signs

1. Hypercarbia (unexplained)
2. Rigidity of the trunk or total body, masseter spasm
3. Tachycardia
4. Tachypnea
5. Unstable blood pressure
6. Mottling
7. Fever
8. Mixed respiratory and metabolic acidosis
9. Myoglobinuria
10. Hyperkalemia
11. Arrhythmias.

If not treated in time, and sometimes even when treated properly, MH can rapidly progress to death. The most common cause of death in this situation is either acute hyperkalemia or disseminated intravascular coagulation from very high body temperature.

Although hyperthermia is one of the main signs of MH, it might not be the first sign. It is extremely important for the anesthesiologist to recognize the early signs of MH, especially an increase in end-tidal carbon dioxide condition. It is also very important to monitor temperature of patients undergoing general anesthesia.

Dantrolene

According to MHAUS, "Dantrolene is the only currently accepted specific treatment for MH".[6] The ryanodine receptor is a dantrolene-binding site. By inhibitory action of dantrolene on this receptor, intracellular release of calcium is decreased, resulting in suppression of the intrinsic mechanism of excitation contraction coupling in the skeletal muscle.[7,8] Dantrolene should be administered as soon as the diagnosis is made. The starting dose is 2.5 mg/kg and it can be repeated up to a cumulative dose of 10 mg/kg. However, if there is no response to higher doses, alternative diagnosis should be considered.

Dantrolene is supplied in 70 ml vials containing 20 mg dantrolene sodium and 3 g mannitol. It is reconstituted with 60 ml sterile water. It is poorly soluble in water and difficulties are experienced in rapidly preparing IV solutions in emergency situations. Thirty-six vials of dantrolene should be available at whatever facility MH triggering agents are used. Dantrolene should be administered by continuous, rapid IV push, preferably via a large vein (but treatment should not be delayed for this reason).

Goals of management in ASC

• *Early recognition of the signs and symptoms*

Educate and update your staff through "in-servicing".

• *Rapid treatment/malignant hyperthermia cart/kit*

Thirty-six vials of dantrolene, sterile water, and other supplies should be present at easily accessible designated locations known by all concerned personnel.

- *Response plan to implement MHAUS-recommended therapies quickly and efficiently*

This plan should be practiced by both the anesthesiologists and nursing staff.

- *Periodic drills*

Review the response program. Frequency of drills at your site may be determined by your staff experience and turnover. However, annual drills should be the minimum according to the Centers for Medicare and Medicaid Services (CMS) in the United States.

Transfer agreement with accepting hospital

Clinical judgment regarding when to transfer a patient should be based on their condition. It is preferable to transfer when stability is evident by the following signs:

1. ETCO$_2$ declining or normal
2. No ominous cardiac dysrhythmias
3. IV dantrolene sodium administration has begun
4. Temperature declining
5. Muscular rigidity is resolving.

In some situations, indicators of stability may not be present with the patient deteriorating rapidly.

Transporting to a nearby, well-equipped hospital instead of continuing stabilization at the ASC may be a better option in such situations. An anesthesiologist should travel in the ambulance with the patient and continue dantrolene administration on the way to hospital.

Transfer arrangements between an ASC and the nearest hospital should be in place. Depending upon your patient population, this hospital should include pediatric or adult critical care setup. According to the MHAUS "Transfer Plan for Suspected MH Patients",[9] this hospital should have the following capabilities:

1. Continuous temperature and cardiopulmonary monitoring.
2. Administration of therapeutic options including non-invasive/invasive cooling, continuous sedation, and antidote therapy (dantrolene by bolus and maintenance therapy, with at least 36 vials available for crisis treatment)
3. Dysrhythmia treatment
4. Hemodialysis

5. Available consultants including anesthesia, critical care, hematology, surgery, nephrology, neurology, and medical toxicology.

Communication with the family

Complications can occur in all phases of medical care. It is important to keep family informed of the situation. The statement should include patient condition, and that the institution has a plan implemented to manage it. If required, the patient will be transferred to another facility.

As soon as the presumptive diagnosis of MH is made, emergency therapy for MH (as described by MHAUS guidelines) should be initiated pending patient transfer to a hospital. One of the key differences in the management of MH in an ambulatory setup as compared with a hospital is limited personnel and resources. Multiple tasks need to be performed at the same time, quickly and efficiently. Assign tasks to your staff, outlined on a worksheet using a checklist format. Responding staff picks up the appropriate worksheet(s) (kept on the MH cart/kit) and performs the tasks outlined.

Checklist for various members of team

I Anesthesiologist

A. Acute phase treatment checklist

1. Signs of MH identified, surgical team informed
2. MH Hotline called: In USA 800-MH-HYPER; outside USA 315-464-7079
3. Initiate treatment
4. Volatile anesthetic agents off and succinylcholine discontinued
5. Hyperventilation with 100% oxygen, high flows (at least >10 l/min)
6. MH cart/kit on the way
7. Instruct surgeon to close/irrigate the wound with cold saline if possible
8. MH cart/kit in room and worksheets distributed
9. Dantrolene being mixed and administered
10. ECG, ETCO$_2$, and core temp continuously monitored
11. Arterial, central, or venous blood gas sent (if possible)
12. K^+, Ca^{2+}, Na^+, and glucose checked (if possible)

13. Hyperkalemia being treated
14. Treating dysrhythmias/ACLS guidelines (do *not* use calcium channel blockers).

B. Cool hyperthermic patient (not lower than 38°C)

1. Cold saline infusion, warming devices off, hypothermia blanket off
2. NG tube in place, lavage with cold saline
3. Wound irrigation
4. Foley catheter placed, urine sample for myoglobinuria obtained, lavage with cold saline if needed
5. Don't overcool.

C. Invasive lines in place if available/needed

D. Labs drawn/ordered

1. CPK
2. Serum myoglobin
3. Urine myoglobin
4. PT/PTT, fibrinogen, FSP, D-Dimer, CBC with platelets
5. Lactic acid
6. Urine output >2 ml/kg/h.

E. Talk to family

F. Transfer arrangements

1. Give detailed report to receiving hospital physician
2. ACLS-level ambulance
3. Accompany the patient.

II Circulator/Scrub nurse

A. Acute phase treatment

1. Bring MH cart/kit, code cart, and defibrillator to crisis area
2. Get material to help close or pack wound
3. Receive worksheet from anesthesia care provider:
    a. Help mix Dantrolene
    b. Prepare and place ice bags to groin and axilla
    c. Place Foley catheter and obtain specimen or begin cold lavage
4. Take telephone worksheet to the secretary/clerk or PACU nurse.

B. After patient is stable

1. Restock supplies on MH cart/kit.

III PACU nurse

A. Acute phase treatment

1. Prepare monitor and bed space for the patient in recovery
2. Ensure defibrillator and code cart are available
3. Offer assistance to OR team
4. Coordinate calling the emergency phone numbers, receiving hospital, ambulance service
5. Record contact person's name and the laboratory (if specimens sent).

B. After patient is stable

1. Confirm receiving hospital is ready
2. Update receiving unit of patient's condition and lines/catheters/monitors.

IV Supply checklist

A. MH cart

1. Dantrolene 36 vials (or equivalent product)
2. Sterile water (without bacteriostatic agent) to dilute Dantrolene
3. 8.4% sodium bicarbonate 50 ml × 2
4. Furosemide 40 mg/ampoule × 2
5. Dextrose (D50) 50 ml vial × 2
6. 10 Calcium Chloride 20 mg vial × 2
7. 2% Lidocaine HCl 20 ml vial × 2
8. 60 ml syringe × 4 to dilute dantrolene
9. IV spike pin × 4 to draw up sterile water for diluting dantrolene
10. IV catheters for IV access and arterial line
11. Nasogastric tubes in various sizes
12. Pressure bag
13. Irrigating syringes × 2 for gastric or bladder irrigation
14. Large plastic bags to fill with ice for patient cooling
15. Bucket for ice
16. AMBU bag for transportation
17. Esophageal temperature probes
18. Arterial and central line transducing equipment
19. D5W 250 ml × 1
20. Microdrip IV set and infusion pump
21. Blood gas kit or 3 ml syringes
22. Specimen tubes for blood/urine.

B. Anesthesia cold supplies in refrigerator

1. 1000 ml normal saline IV × 3
2. Regular insulin 100 u/ml x 1.

C. Nursing supplies

1. Large sterile adhesive drape to cover wound
2. Three-way irrigating Foley catheters in multiple sizes
3. 60 ml Toomy-type irrigating syringe × 2
4. Large plastic bags for ice
5. Small plastic bags for ice
6. Container for ice.

Management of MH-susceptible patient

Malignant hyperthermia-susceptible patients can be safely anesthetized at ambulatory centers using non-triggering agents.[1,7] The anesthesia machine should be prepared according to the manufacturer's recommendations. ETCO$_2$ and temperature monitoring is critical. After an uneventful anesthetic, prolonged monitoring in PACU is not required. Discharge instructions should include the recommendation of g oing to hospital if temperature elevation or dark-colored urine is noted.

References

1. Denborough MA, Forster JFA, Lovell RRH, Maplestone PA, Villiers JD: Anaesthetic deaths in a family. *Brit J Anaesth* 1962; 34: 395–396.
2. Rosero EB, Adesanya AO, Timaran CH, Joshi GP: Trends and outcomes of malignant hyperthermia in the United States, 2000 to 2005. *Anesthesiology* 2009; 110:89–94.
3. Gillard E, Otsu K, Fujii J et al: A substitution of cysteine for arginine 614 in the ryanodine receptor is potentially causative of human malignant hyperthermia. *Genomics* 1991;11(3):751–755.
4. Galli L, Orrico A, Lorenzini et al: Frequency and localization of mutations in the 106 exons of the RYR1 gene in 50 individuals with malignant hyperthermia. *Hum Mutat* 2006; 27(8):830.
5. Krause T, Gerbeshagen MU, Fiege M et al: Dantrolene – A review of its pharmacology, therapeutic use and new developments. *Anaesthesia* 2004; 59(4):364–373.
6. Litman RS: Management of MH and MH-Susceptible Patients in the Ambulatory Setting, ASA refresher course lecture at 2010 ASA Annual Meeting.
7. Malignant Hyperthermia Association of the United States. *MHAUS Transfer of Care Guidelines*, 2015.

Delayed emergence

Claude Abdallah

Introduction

Delayed emergence is a major concern for the anesthesiologist. A patient with delayed awakening from anesthesia must be approached in a systemic fashion, using medical history, clinical findings, and laboratory evaluation to rapidly diagnose and appropriately manage the most likely cause. In most cases, causes of delayed emergence can be quickly identified by clinical context. Different etiologies may be responsible for delayed awakening in a patient, with the most common etiologies classified as pharmacological, metabolic, or neurological causes.

Educational objectives

1. Describe major etiologies of delayed emergence
2. Take steps to manage delayed emergence
3. Discuss measures to prevent delayed emergence

Scenario 1: Narcotic over-sedation

You are called urgently to assess a patient post general anesthesia secondary to increased breathing effort with oxygen saturation in the mid 80s and lengthy emergence from anesthesia. The patient is a 6-year-old boy, who underwent tonsillectomy and adenoidectomy.

Expected actions:

1. Airway support and ventilation/ supplemental oxygenation
2. Call for help if needed
3. Evaluate hemodynamic status
4. Evaluate level of consciousness
5. Assess muscle tonus/strength

6. Obtain more information regarding the intraoperative anesthesia management.

Scenario continued:

The patient is hemodynamically stable, there is no blood suctioned from the oral cavity. Patient is opening eyes when stimulated with improvement of oxygen saturation, but goes back to sleep with slow respiratory rate and airway obstruction when left alone. Patient has a medical history significant for obesity, obstructive sleep apnea, and situational anxiety. Family history is non-contributory. The review of anesthesia chart showed that oral midazolam was administered as premedication, an uneventful mask induction with O_2/ N_2O/sevoflurane, with easy endotracheal intubation after IV administration of propofol 3 mg/kg and morphine 0.15 mg/kg. Patient's trachea was extubated deep at the end of procedure that lasted 45 min, with blow-by supplemental oxygen.

Expected actions:

1. Continue supporting airway/supplemental oxygenation
2. Reassure the patient, constantly
3. Consider reversal of narcotics/sedation.

Scenario continued:

Spontaneous respiratory rate is 5 breaths/min. Pupils are equally constricted bilaterally, faint bilateral breath sounds are heard on chest auscultation. Patient becomes more responsive with IV titration of naloxone (0.3 mcg/kg/dose), respiratory rate increases to 14 breaths/min, with normalization of oxygen saturation without airway support.

Perioperative Drill-Based Crisis Management, ed. Steven Butz. Published by Cambridge University Press. © Cambridge University Press 2016.

Expected actions:

1. Arrange for overnight admission to a monitored bed/ICU
2. Debrief family and care team
3. Schedule for a follow-up on the next day.

Debriefing

- Identify two or three things the team felt went well with the scenario.
- Identify two or three things the team felt they should have done differently.
- Is staff familiar with administration (dose/contraindications) of reversal agents for different medications used routinely in your practice?
- Are these reversal medications easy to find?
- Is hospital admission on an emergency basis easily initiated in your facility?
- Identify up to three process improvements the facility will develop after the drill that will better equip them for next time.

Discussion

Pharmacological causes of delayed emergence can be correlated with timing, total dose, half-life, protein binding, and metabolism or clearance of anesthetic drugs. In addition to their direct sedative effect, administration of narcotics results in respiratory depression by decreasing response to hypercarbia, causing hypoventilation with slow breathing or apneic pauses and subsequent decreased clearance of volatile agents. Severe hypercapnia is often associated and contributes to residual narcosis.

Recurrent hypoxemia in young children with obstructive sleep apnea is associated with increased analgesic sensitivity to opiates and reduced opioid requirement for analgesia (1,2). This becomes more severe in obese patients when opioids are administered based on measured body weight. Some literature recommends that opioids when used are titrated to spontaneous ventilation whenever possible (3).

The priority in the management is to support the airway and ventilation, suctioning the patient's airway if needed. Observe and auscultate the chest, for wheezing or rales. Assess circulation. In an arousable patient, assess patient's strength by hand grip and sustained head lift if neuromuscular blockade has been used. Paradoxical respirations suggest airway obstruction or inadequate reversal of neuromuscular blockade.

Reversal of opioids may be necessary if the patient is hypoventilating. However, reversal of side effects (respiratory depression, CNS depression) by using naloxone (pure opioid antagonist with a greater affinity for the mu-opioid receptor) may be associated with severe pain and agitation. Therefore, if the patient is otherwise stable, and assisted ventilation is adequate, naloxone is better titrated in a controlled setting while insuring adequate ventilatory support. The onset time of naloxone is 1–2 min, and duration is dose dependent. Risk of "remorphinization" is always possible, most opioids having a longer duration of action than naloxone, and therefore prolonged follow-up is recommended. Continuous infusion of naloxone may be required and adjusted to clinical response.

Naloxone can be administered by diluting one vial IV (400 mcg in 1 ml) in 9 ml normal saline. In adults, 20–40 mcg (0.5–1 ml) is administered IV and titrated to effect. Naloxone may be administered via many routes, including IV, intraosseous, intramuscular, intratracheal, and subcutaneous. For children who are ventilating but in whom opioid-induced respiratory depression necessitates antagonism in the perioperative period, it is reasonable to titrate naloxone IV in small doses of 0.25 to 0.5 mcg/kg IV, until improvement of ventilation. Some literature suggests that in order to ensure that recrudescence of the respiratory depression does not occur, the same cumulative total IV dose of naloxone is administered subsequently as an intramuscular injection.

Allergy to naloxone has been described. Increased sympathetic activity, profound systemic hypertension, cardiac arrhythmias (including ventricular fibrillation), and pulmonary edema (noncardiogenic) have been reported with overzealous dosing of naloxone. Pulmonary edema may occur and may not be a dose-dependent side effect to naloxone (4), since it has been reported after conservative doses.

Reversal of hypnotic and sedative effects of benzodiazepines may be achieved with flumazenil. In adults, 0.2 mg is administered IV (over 15 s) and titrated (0.2 mg/min) to a maximum of 1 mg in 5 min, 3 mg in 1 h. Higher cumulative doses may be required in divided doses or as infusion in some cases of benzodiazepine overdose. Since the duration of action of flumazenil is shorter than that of most benzodiazepines, reoccurrence of sedation is possible and patients should be monitored for maintenance of reversal, with repeat doses (0.2 mg q 20 min prn) or IV infusion of flumazenil (0.2–0.4 mg/h), if needed. For pediatric dosage: Initial: 0.01mg/kg (up to 0.2mg) IV of flumazenil over 15 s; titrate: Further injection of 0.01 mg/kg/min where necessary, up to a max of four additional doses, until desired level of consciousness is obtained. Max total dose: 0.05 mg/kg or 1 mg, whichever is lower. Dizziness, nausea/vomiting, increased sweating, headache, abnormal or blurred vision, cardiac dysrhythmias, agitation, and injection site pain may occur with flumazenil administration. Flumazenil has been associated with seizures, most frequently in patients who have either been on long-term benzodiazepines or with cyclic antidepressant overdose.

Scenario 2: Prolonged neuromuscular blockade

A 6-year-old, healthy child is scheduled for an esophagogastroduodenoscopy/colonoscopy secondary to gastroesophageal reflux and vomiting. Propofol (3 mg/kg), succinylcholine (1 mg/kg), and fentanyl (1 mcg/kg) were administered IV prior to intubation. There is a change of provider from the anesthesia team toward the end of the case. Twenty minutes after conclusion of the procedure, the patient is still intubated with no evidence of spontaneous respirations.

Expected actions:

1. Continue airway support and ventilation
2. Check hemodynamic stability and temperature
3. Confirm that all IV and inhalational anesthetic agents are off
4. Check for residual muscular paralysis
5. Perform neurological exam if possible: pupils, presence, or absence of gag/cough, symmetric motor movement
6. Reassess and eliminate medication administration error
7. Call for help if needed.

Scenario continued:

There was no response to peripheral nerve stimulation.

Expected actions:

1. Administer light sedation to prevent awareness

2. Verify family history of anesthesia "allergies" or complications
3. Reconfirm that no additional muscle relaxants were administered
4. Consider drawing a plasma cholinesterase (PChE) level and a dibucaine number.

Scenario continued:

Twenty minutes later, the patient started to breathe spontaneously. The gastroenterologist is requesting to speed up the turnover of the room so he can meet his clinic schedule.

Expected actions:

1. Verify that the patient is breathing spontaneously with adequate tidal volumes
2. Stop sedation and assess muscular tonus and strength
3. Keep the airway secure and the patient monitored until full recovery of muscle relaxation
4. Call for help if needed
5. Communicate the patient's recovery status with OR care team involved
6. Consider moving the patient, if stable and under close monitoring, intubated and lightly sedated if possible.

Scenario continued:

Suspecting a residual neuromuscular blockade, the covering anesthesiologist administers a reversal dose of neostigmine/glycopyrrolate, the trachea is extubated and the patient transferred with O_2 face mask assistance. A few minutes later, the patient experiences a sudden decrease in O_2 saturation and a call for a stat anesthesia help is initiated. The patient appears hypotonic, with very faint breathing efforts.

Expected actions:

1. Airway support and ventilation/supplemental oxygenation/consider ETT placement with sedation
2. Evaluate hemodynamic status and resuscitate if needed, continue charting vital signs
3. Evaluate level of consciousness, consider depth of anesthesia monitor
4. Assess muscle tonus/strength
5. Reassure the patient, constantly.

Table 4.1 Evoked responses during depolarizing (phases I and II) and non-depolarizing block

Evoked stimulus	Depolarizing block		Non-depolarizing block
	Phase I	Phase II	
Train-of-four	Constant but diminished	Fade	Fade
Tetany	Constant but diminished	Fade	Fade
Double-burst stimulation	Constant but diminished	Fade	Fade
Post-tetanic potentiation	Absent	Present	Present

Scenario continued:

Airway was supported with endotracheal intubation, and the trachea was extubated two hours later after verification of adequate muscle strength (clinically and by peripheral nerve stimulation) with uneventful recovery.

Expected actions:

1. Schedule a follow-up with the family.

Debriefing

- Identify two or three things the team felt went well with the scenario.
- Identify two or three things the team felt they should have done differently.
- Is staff familiar with assessing and managing prolonged muscular recovery associated with delayed emergence?
- Is handling more than a routine laboratory specimen easily initiated in your facility?
- Was there any problem with communication between the different care teams, and how can this be improved? Are there guidelines for PACU and OR cases sign out in your facility?
- Is there difficulty in having functional equipment such as nerve stimulators readily available in operating rooms in your facility?
- Are there clear guidelines in your facility about the possibility of care of an intubated and sedated patient outside of the operating room, such as in the recovery room?
- Identify up to three process improvements the facility will develop after the drill that will better equip them for next time.

Discussion

Several factors may contribute to postoperative residual paralysis and prolong muscle relaxants effects, including delay in metabolism and clearance, inadequacy of reversal, acidosis, electrolyte imbalance, hypothermia, and interaction with other drugs (5). The patient appears hypotonic with poorly coordinated respiratory muscle activity. The patient is unable to sustain a head lift or hand grasp. In infants and children, return of muscle tone and/or depth of respirations to preoperative status is assessed. Weakness of the pharyngeal muscles may result in upper airway collapse with airway obstruction after tracheal extubation. Hypoventilation resulting from residual neuromuscular blockade should be treated rapidly with ventilatory support, patient reassurance, and sedation if needed until resolution of residual neuromuscular blockade. Reversal agents are supplemented in divided doses up to dose limitations. See Table 4.1 for expected responses to evoked response testing. Sugammadex (ORG 25969) is a relatively new reversal agent, effective in antagonizing rocuronium rapidly after the onset of neuromuscular blockade. It encapsulates rocuronium and prevents further action of rocuronium. To date, sugammadex is not available for clinical use in the United States, but is in countries throughout the world.

Paradoxical weakness may result from excessive reversal agent administration. Reversal agents are of no benefit in reversing a depolarizing block. By increasing neuromuscular junction acetylcholine concentration and inhibiting pseudocholinesterase, cholinesterase inhibitors prolong depolarization blockade. Pseudocholinesterase (PChE), also known as plasma cholinesterase, is a serine hydrolase capable of hydrolyzing esters including acetylcholine, succinylcholine, mivacurium, and ester-type local anesthetics such as procaine, chloroprocaine, tetracaine, cocaine, and heroin. Two types of serum cholinesterase exist: a normal and an atypical variety. Both types are genetically transmitted. About 95% of the population carry only the normal esterase (homozygous), about 4% a mixture of both enzymes (heterozygous), and about 1 in 2800 (0.04%) the atypical

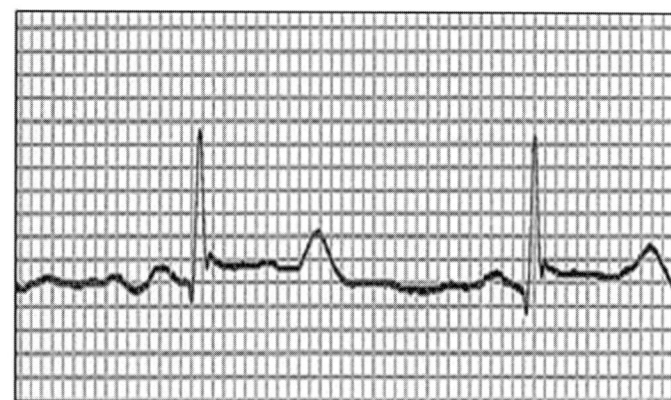

Figure 4.1 Osborn wave

esterase (homozygous) (6,7). Low pseudocholinesterase level may mean a reduced amount of the normal enzyme or the presence of the atypical enzyme in varying amounts. Qualitative tests, dibucaine number, and fluoride number reflect a reduction in PChE resulting from the addition of dibucaine or sodium fluoride to the assay. Dibucaine (nupercaine), a local anesthetic, will inhibit the activity of the normal enzyme to a greater extent than the atypical one, irrespective of the actual plasma levels of either. It inhibits normal pseudocholinesterase activity by 80%, but inhibits the homozygous atypical enzyme by only 20%. The heterozygous enzyme is characterized by an intermediate 40–60% inhibition. The percentage of inhibition of pseudocholinesterase activity is termed the dibucaine number. The dibucaine number is proportional to pseudocholinesterase function and is independent of the amount of enzyme. Therefore adequacy of pseudocholinesterase can be determined quantitatively in the laboratory, in units per liter, and qualitatively by the dibucaine number (8,9). Results for evoked responses for muscle relaxants can be seen in Table 4.1.

Scenario 3: Hypothermia in the recovery room

A 38-year-old, healthy, athletic female patient with a history of severe nausea/vomiting after anesthesia is scheduled for breast reduction under general anesthesia. Total IV anesthesia was administered to prevent postoperative nausea and vomiting, with an IV infusion of propofol, dexmedetomidine, fentanyl, and acetaminophen. Three hours later and at the conclusion of the surgery, the trachea was extubated deep with a respiratory rate of 6 bpm

and a heart rate of 40 bpm. Upon transfer to the stretcher, the patient became apneic with a heart rate of 35 bpm.

Expected actions:

1. Establish airway support and ventilation
2. Assess hemodynamics/rhythm and pulse
3. Apply ACLS bradycardia algorithm
4. Treat etiology of bradycardia
5. Confirm that all anesthetic agents are off
6. Reassess and confirm dosage and medications used, including reversal agents
7. Check for residual muscular paralysis
8. Perform neurological exam if possible: pupils, presence or absence of gag/cough, symmetric motor movement
9. Rule out CO_2 narcosis
10. Check patient's temperature
11. Call for help if needed.

Scenario continued:

Patient is still requiring ventilatory support, despite all IV anesthetics being stopped. Blood loss was 300 ml, and patient had received 2.5 l of lactated Ringer's (LR) during the procedure. Total IV narcotics given were verified as adequate. Osborn waves (J point elevation of QT with prominent notching of the terminal portion of QRS) are noticed on the ECG in Figure 4.1. Fluid warmer was not used during the case. Temperature probe was disconnected during the last part of the procedure for dressing application in a beach chair position. Patient temperature is confirmed at 32.5°C. The lower body forced-air warmer was found to be set at ambient temperature (instead of 38°C) for a good part of the case.

Expected actions:

1. Call for help, if needed
2. Secure airway and ventilation
3. Actively warm the patient; increase OR temperature
4. Reverse neuromuscular blockade if present, after rewarming
5. Administer sedation, if needed, to prevent awareness
6. Prevent and treat shivering
7. Debrief family
8. Debrief surgery team.

Scenario continued:

After rewarming, the patient was able to open her eyes and have purposeful movements. Osborn waves disappeared after 4 h of PACU stay. Recovery course was reassessed and was uneventful.

Debriefing

- Identify two or three things the team felt went well with the scenario.
- Identify two or three things the team felt they should have done differently.
- Is there difficulty in circulating in the operating rooms (i.e. to the feet of the patient) in order to assess bleeding, positioning, functioning of equipment (such as patient warming system) or in order to perform resuscitation?
- Are cognitive aids available and used?
- Did the team react quickly to help? Were there any communication problems between the different members of the team?
- Identify up to three process improvements the facility will develop after the drill that will better equip them for next time.

Discussion

General anesthesia increases the temperature inter-threshold range 20-fold (from 0.2 to 4°C): a broad temperature range over which active thermoregulatory responses are absent and patients are poikilothermic. The effects of anesthesia medications on thermoregulation are diverse, including central effect on hypothalamus, inhibition of brown fat thermogenesis, vasoconstriction, and vasodilation. Major mechanisms of heat loss in the OR are radiation (infrared electromagnetic waves), convection, evaporation, and conduction. Effects of hypothermia include vasoconstriction with increase in systemic vascular resistance (SVR) and CVP, a decrease in renal blood flow and glomerular filtration with cold diuresis, impaired coagulation and a leftward shift of oxyhemoglobin dissociation curve, as well as an increase in wound infections and an increase in duration of hospitalization. Hypothermia decreases response to hypercapnia, increases solubility of volatile agents, increases protein binding, and reduces rate of biotransformation and clearance of medications with prolonged neuromuscular blockade. Hypothermia delays the discharge from PACU and may prolong the need for ventilatory support. Shivering increases the baseline metabolic rate, and increases wound pain and intraocular and intracranial pressures. Patients should remain intubated until awake and close to normothermic.

Electrocardiographic abnormalities associated with hypothermia include Osborn waves, prolonged PR and QT intervals, sinus bradycardia, atrial and ventricular dysrhythmias, and shivering artifacts. Hypothermia induces a difference between epicardial and endocardial potassium channel currents. Osborn waves are the electrocardiographic reflection of the transmural voltage gradient, and may persist after resumption of normothermia. The differential diagnosis would include normal variant of early repolarization, hypercalcemia, CNS lesions, coronary vasospasm, LVH, Brugada syndrome, and drug abuse (10).

Prevention of hypothermia includes covering the patient; increasing the operating room temperature; using a warming mattress, forced air warmer, thermal cap, heating pad, infrared heater, IV fluid/ blood warmer, and warm lavage solution; humidification and warming of inspired gases; and use of low-flow anesthesia.

Scenario 4: Metablolic derangement in recovery room

A 14-month-old, ex-premature (born at 26 weeks PCA) child, scheduled for bilateral inguinal hernia repair and circumcision, is moved to your staffed OR room in the afternoon. There was unexpected delay in surgical cases in other operating rooms. Patient has developmental delay, GERD, mild hypotonia, and a history of seizures at birth. Anti-seizure medications have been stopped last month because of absence of occurrence of seizures. Patient received general anesthesia with caudal block using ropivacaine 0.2% 0.8 ml/kg. Thirty minutes after the end of the surgery, the patient is still apneic.

Expected actions:

1. Continue airway support and ventilation
2. Assess hemodynamics/rhythm and pulse
3. Confirm that all anesthetic agents are off
4. Reassess and confirm dosage and medications used, including reversal agents
5. Check for residual muscular paralysis
6. Perform neurological exam if possible: pupils, presence or absence of gag/cough, symmetric motor movement
7. Rule out CO_2 narcosis
8. Rule out a high level of regional blockade
9. Check patient's temperature
10. Call for help if needed.

Scenario continued:

Patient has stable hemodynamics. Esophageal temperature is 36.5°C. All anesthesia medications have been verified as adequately administered to the weight of the patient, no paralytic agent was used. Lactated Ringer's (25 ml/kg) was administered during the case. Blood loss was minimal. Caudal block was easily performed with negative aspiration. With painful stimulation, patient is moving four extremities. Diffuse tremors/shaking are noticed with increase in blood pressure and tachycardia.

Expected actions:

1. Continue supporting airway and breathing
2. Measure blood glucose level/point-of-care glucose test STAT
3. Administer glucose bolus
4. Assess and treat for seizures
5. Check arterial blood gas, lactate, and electrolytes
6. Request neurology consult
7. Call for help if needed.

Scenario continued:

Patient's blood glucose level was 30 mg/dl. Patient received midazolam (0.1/mg/kg/IV) and a D50% 1 ml/kg IV bolus.

Expected actions:

1. Repeat blood glucose measurement

2. Start glucose infusion
3. Consider endocrinology consult (to rule out metabolic disorders)
4. Prepare for overnight admission.

Scenario continued:

Neurology and endocrinology team were consulted and airway was secured with patient sedated until stabilization and recovery to baseline status. Patient was admitted for overnight stay with close monitoring.

Expected actions:

1. Debrief the family
2. Arrange for follow-up of patient/family
3. Discuss guidelines for IV placement or clear fluid administration after a prolonged NPO time in your facility.

Debriefing

- Identify two or three things the team felt went well with the scenario.
- Identify two or three things the team felt they should have done differently.
- Are there guidelines for IV placement or clear fluid administration after a prolonged NPO time in your facility?
- Is the staff familiar with metabolic disease and electrolyte abnormalities associated with long recovery?
- Is glucose and blood gas analysis readily available and easily performed in your facility?
- Is consulting other subspecialties (endocrinology/neurology, etc.) or hospital admission on an emergency basis easily done in your facility?
- Identify up to three process improvements the facility will develop after the drill that will better equip them for next time.

Discussion

Central nervous system (CNS) depression may occur with multiple systemic metabolic disturbances. This may increase the sensitivity to CNS depressants and appear as residual anesthetic effect with delayed emergence and recovery from anesthesia. In an ambulatory surgical care setting, these problems result mostly from an undiagnosed pathology or patient noncompliance to therapy.

The stress of anesthesia and surgery usually causes increased blood glucose levels. However, hypoglycemia may occur in diabetic patients, or after manipulation of insulin-producing tumors and retroperitoneal carcinomas. Pediatric patients are at increased risk for hypoglycemia, especially neonates and preterm infants, infants of diabetic mothers, or small for gestational age, or those with erythroblastosis fetalis. Also, children in the lower percentiles of weight, those with chronic debilitating illness, or those who have been receiving total parenteral nutrition are vulnerable to hypoglycemia. Extensive preoperative fasting increases the risk of hypoglycemia and should be avoided or managed with IV/PO fluid supplementation. Acute treatment of suspected or known hypoglycemia consists of administering dextrose (glucose) IV/IO at 0.5–1 g/kg. D50W: 1–2ml/kg IV/IO bolus, or D25W: 2–4 ml/kg IV/IO bolus, or D10W: 5–10 ml/kg IV/IO bolus and dextrose 10% IV infusion at 1–2 ml/kg/h.

Hyperosmolar hyperglycemic nonketotic coma would be extremely rare in ambulatory care, because of its association with severe conditions (sepsis, pancreatitis, pneumonia, uremia, burns, and administration of hypertonic solutions or mannitol). Adrenal insufficiency is associated with prolonged unconsciousness after anesthesia. Hypo-osmolarity, as seen in hyponatremia, is often caused by dilution after absorption of large volumes during transurethral resection of the prostate, or by the syndrome of inappropriate antidiuretic hormone secretion. Other electrolyte disorders such as hypercalcemia, hypocalcemia, hypomagnesemia, and hypernatremia may be responsible for prolonged postoperative emergence.

Hypothyroid patients have a diminished cardiac output, decreased intravascular volume, and blunted baroreceptor reflexes and are more susceptible to the hypotensive effect of anesthetic agents. The coexistence of primary adrenal insufficiency or congestive heart failure should be considered in cases of refractory hypotension. Associated problems with hypothyroidism include hypoglycemia, anemia, hyponatremia, and hypothermia from a low basal metabolic rate. Recovery from general anesthesia may be delayed in hypothyroid patients by decrease drug biotransformation, hypothermia, and respiratory depression.

Scenario 5: Intraoperative Stroke

A 68-year-old male with medical history of hypertension and non-insulin-dependent diabetes and a full, large beard presents for a cervical node excision. He received midazolam IV preoperatively, followed by general anesthesia with IV propofol, fentanyl, and rocuronium and maintained with sevoflurane in O_2 and air. The procedure was more prolonged and more extensive than scheduled, with moderate intraoperative bleeding and controlled hemodynamic instability. At the end of the procedure, and after surgical dressing application, the patient's oxygen saturation suddenly dropped.

Expected actions:

1. Assume hypoxemia
2. Airway support and ventilation/supplemental oxygenation
3. Check that ventilation is adequate
4. Check vital signs
5. Call for help if needed.

Scenario continued:

The endotracheal tube was noticed to have been accidentally dislodged. Patient was noted to be difficult to ventilate with 100% O_2 and positive pressure. After two-hands mask technique, followed by succinylcholine and increasing inhalation anesthesia, hypotension was noted.

Expected actions:

1. Call for help, if needed, and difficult airway cart
2. Ensure adequate oxygenation and ventilation
3. Check vital signs
4. Turn down/off anesthetics
5. Expand blood volume
6. Consider vasopressors
7. Elucidate and correct cause of hypotension.

Scenario continued:

A large neck hematoma is noted with increased difficulty in ventilating, followed by a cardiac arrest with asystole.

Expected actions:

1. Initiate CPR and ACLS treatment for asystole
2. Call for difficult airway cart
3. Call for surgery.

Scenario continued:

Patient's trachea was successfully intubated and patient was resuscitated while surgeon explored the surgical field and controlled hemostasis. At the end of the procedure, patient was breathing spontaneously, but stayed unresponsive to physical stimulation.

Expected actions:

1. Ensure adequate oxygenation and ventilation
2. Confirm that all inhalational and intravenous anesthetic agents are off
3. Check for residual muscular paralysis with nerve stimulator and reverse neuromuscular blockade as appropriate. Check patient's temperature and warm, if necessary
4. Perform neurological exam if possible: pupils, symmetric motor movement, presence or absence of gag/cough
5. If available, check arterial blood gas, electrolytes, and blood glucose level, and treat if needed.

Scenario continued:

Patient has abnormal neurological exam and response to painful stimuli. Blood glucose level and electrolytes are within normal limits and reversal of neuromuscular blockade is appropriate with no residual inhalation or intravenous agents on board. Axillary temperature is 35.5°C.

Expected actions:

1. Inform the surgeon
2. Obtain an urgent neurology or neurosurgery consult
3. Maintain hemodynamic stability
4. Arrange for transfer and a stat head CT scan
5. Prepare to transfer the patient to ICU with close neurology follow-up.

Debriefing

- Identify two or three things the team felt went well with the scenario.
- Identify two or three things the team felt they should have done differently.
- Is staff familiar with possible postoperative neurological complications and able to manage them?
- Is consulting other subspecialties (neurology) or hospital admission on an urgent basis easily done in your facility?
- Identify up to three process improvements the facility will develop after the drill which will better equip them for next time.

Discussion

The workup for delayed emergence starts usually with the most common reasons. After considering residual anesthetic effects in a patient who experiences delayed emergence, a rapid check of the other common causes is undertaken such as increased sensitivity to anesthesia medications (age, drug interactions, renal or hepatic disease, obesity …); delay in arousal may also result from hypercarbia, hypothermia, and metabolic pathologies. Other causes are hypoxic brain injury, or neurological insult such as ischemia/hemorrhagic stroke, acute increase in intracranial pressure, or undetected head injury. After ruling out residual drug effects, if decreased awareness persists beyond a reasonable period of observation, with normal serum glucose, arterial blood gases, and electrolyte values, CNS etiologies must be considered. Postictal status may be considered in a patient with seizure history.

Cerebral hypoperfusion may be caused by reduced cardiac output, occlusive cerebrovascular disease, or decreased systemic vascular resistance (shock). Hypotension occurring perioperatively may result in cerebral ischemia, and stroke and is more frequent in patients with preoperative cerebrovascular disease. Arterial compression from improper positioning or retraction of the head and neck are other causes of hypoperfusion. Thromboembolic events may occur in patients undergoing cardiac, vascular, and invasive neck procedures, or in patients with atrial fibrillation or hypercoagulable states. Venous air embolus is possible in cases where positioning of the surgical site is higher than the heart; even small amounts of air are dangerous in patients with R–L cardiac shunts. Paradoxical air embolism is a major risk in patients with probe-patent foramen ovale.

Hypertension is a frequent cause of cerebral hyperperfusion. It may lead to stroke via hemorrhage and increased intracranial pressure (ICP) with compression and possible herniation of brain tissue. ICP may increase during hyperperfusion, intracerebral or subdural hemorrhage or hematoma, cerebral edema, pneumocephalus, or malfunctioning ventriculoperitoneal shunt.

In cases of neurological complications, a neurology/neurosurgery consult and radiological imaging of the CNS should be obtained as soon as possible, in order to start appropriate management.

References

1. Brown KA, Laferrière A, Lakheeram I, Moss IR. Recurrent hypoxemia in children is associated with increased analgesic sensitivity to opiates. *Anesthesiology* 2006; 105(4):665–669.

2. Brown KA, Laferrière A, Moss IR. Recurrent hypoxemia in young children with obstructive sleep apnea is associated with reduced opioid requirement for analgesia. *Anesthesiology* 2004; 100(4):806–810.

3. Lerman J, Cote CJ, Steward DJ. *Manual of Pediatric Anesthesia*. 6th edition. Churchill Livingstone. Chapter 10: Otorhinolaryngology. p. 286.

4. Prough DS, Roy R, Bumgarner J, Shannon G. Acute pulmonary edema in healthy teenagers following conservative doses of intravenous naloxone. *Anesthesiology* 1984; 60:485–486.

5. Srivastava A, Hunter JM. Reversal of neuromuscular block. *Br J Anaesth* 2009; 103(1): 115–129.

6. Pantuck EJ. Plasma cholinesterase: Gene and variations. *Anesth Analg* 1993; 77:380–386.

7. Jensen FS, Shwartz M, Viby-Mogensen J. Identification of human plasma cholinesterase variants using molecular biological techniques. *Acta Anaesthesiol Scand* 1995; 39:142–149.

8. Levano S, Ginz H, Siegemund M, Filipovic M, Voronkov E, Urwyler A, Girard T. Genotyping the butyrylcholinesterase in patients with prolonged neuromuscular block after succinylcholine. *Anesthesiology* 2005; 102: 531–535.

9. Cerf C, Mesguish M, Gabriel I, Amselem S, Duvaldestin P. Screening patients with prolonged neuromuscular blockade after succinylcholine and mivacurium. *Anesth Analg* 2002; 94(2):461–466.

10. Vassallo SU, Delaney KA, Hoffman RS, Slater W, Goldfrank LR. A prospective evaluation of the electrocardiographic manifestations of hypothermia. *Acad Emerg Med* 1999; 6:1121–1126.

Recovery room issues

Rose Campise-Luther

Introduction

The incidence of perioperative complications is increased in the immediate postoperative period. Production pressure and the reduced acuity of the Ambulatory Surgery Center (ASC) patient population can lead to an earlier transfer of patients to the PACU, at a time when they are most vulnerable.

This chapter will present three case scenarios of events that can be encountered in the PACU.

Educational objectives

1. Appropriately identify symptoms of potentially life-threatening events in the PACU
2. Prioritize the differential diagnosis of these symptoms according to their risk potential and severity
3. Correctly identify the treatment pathway for potentially life-threatening events.

Scenario 1: Postoperative upper airway obstruction

A 17-year-old male presents to the PACU after an uneventful right knee arthroscopy with removal of a loose body and repair of a meniscal tear. He has a history of obesity (BMI: 43), obstructive sleep apnea (OSA), and metabolic syndrome. He underwent a general endotracheal anesthetic and received 30 mg ketorolac and 200 mcg fentanyl intraoperatively for pain. His oxygen saturation (SpO_2) on 2 l of oxygen via nasal cannula is 91%. Shortly after the transfer of care his SpO_2 drops to 87%.

Expected actions:

1. Call for help if needed

2. Assess patient consciousness and respiratory effort
3. Ensure oxygen supply/availability of bag mask
4. Change to non-rebreather mask with an FiO_2 of 1.0.

Scenario continued:

The patient is unconscious, as he had been extubated deep and transferred to the PACU quickly. His other vital signs are as follows: heart rate (HR) 98, blood pressure (BP) 162/98, respiratory rate (RR) 19. Although there is respiratory effort, no air movement or sound is detected on ausculation.

Expected actions:

1. Attempt to establish an airway via head tilt/ jaw thrust
2. Use assisted ventilation with bag mask and an inspired oxygen concentration of 1.0
3. If needed, use two-person mask ventilation.

Scenario continued:

Although the patient is squirming with the airway manipulation, there is still no air movement. You are able to positive pressure ventilate. The SpO_2 improves to 90%.

Expected actions:

1. Continue assisted ventilation
2. Consider airway adjuncts
3. Place patient in lateral position.

Scenario continued:

The drill ends with the insertion of a nasal trumpet and establishment of a patent airway and improvement of oxygen saturation.

Perioperative Drill-Based Crisis Management, ed. Steven Butz. Published by Cambridge University Press. © Cambridge University Press 2016.

Scenario 2: Hyperthermia in recovery room

A 53-year-old female presents to the PACU after a left knee arthroscopy with meniscus repair. The case had been scheduled for 45 min, but took 153 min secondary to technical difficulties. The patient has a history of obesity, hyperthyroidism, gastroesophageal reflux, and postoperative nausea and vomiting. The anesthesiologist reports that she required intubation after unsuccessful attempts to place an LMA. She received two doses of succinylcholine for a difficult intubation and glycopyrrolate for bradycardia. Upon arrival in the PACU the patient is asleep and her vital signs are HR 136, BP 150/97, RR 32, SpO_2 95% on room air, axillary temperature 38.9°C. The patient is flushed and perspiring.

Expected actions:

1. Assess consciousness and respiratory status of patient
2. Remove coverings
3. Monitor EKG and temperature closely.

Scenario continued:

The patient is incoherent and agitated. The repeat vitals are HR 145, BP 165/99, RR 40, SpO_2 93% on room air, axillary temperature 39.1°C. The EKG monitor shows a highly irregular rhythm.

Expected actions:

1. Call for help
2. Consider active cooling
3. Review patient history and anesthetic
4. Consider differential diagnosis and prioritize according to risk potential (iatrogenic, malignant hyperthermia, neuroleptic malignant syndrome, infectious, anticholinergic medications)
5. Determine rhythm and need for intervention.

Scenario continued:

The anesthesiologist returns to the bedside. The rhythm is determined to be atrial fibrillation. Ice packs are being placed in the neck area of the patient and her HR initially slows to 92, only to return to 148 shortly thereafter. Her BP is 110/62, SpO_2 93% on room air, axillary temperature 39.2°C.

Expected actions:

1. Administer fluid bolus
2. Continue active cooling

3. Consider administration of a beta-blocker or calcium channel blocker for rate control.

Scenario continued:

Before a beta-blocker can be administered, the patient starts seizing.

Expected actions:

1. Protect patient from harm by placing a bite block and rail cushions
2. Administer lorazepam IV (or other benzodiazepine)
3. Continue to cool the patient
4. Administer NSAIDs for further temperature control.

Scenario continued:

The patient stops seizing. The EKG shows persistent atrial fibrillation. HR 145, BP 120/95, oxygen saturation 93%, axillary temperature 39°C.

Expected actions:

1. Consider using beta-blocker or calcium channel blocker for rate control
2. Consider starting anti-thyroid medications should these be available
3. Make arrangements to transfer patient to an affiliated acute care hospital.

Scenario continued:

The drill ends when the HR is controlled, the vital signs continue to be stable, and the patient is transferred via ambulance to an acute care hospital accompanied by the anesthesiologist.

Scenario 3: Postoperative dysrhythmia

A 73-year-old male is admitted to the PACU after undergoing closed reduction of a nasal fracture. He has history of coronary artery disease s/p myocardial infarction at age 67 and balloon dilatation at that time. He is currently asymptomatic with reasonable exercise tolerance on a diuretic and digoxin. The patient had undergone an uneventful general anesthetic with sevoflurane, dolasetron, and fentanyl. In the PACU his initial vital signs are HR 165, initial BP 145/75, SpO_2 on room air 93%, axillary temperature 35.7°C.

Expected actions:

1. Evaluate patient, level of consciousness, respiratory status, level of discomfort

2. Provide warm blankets or other means of active warming.

Scenario continued:

The patient is becoming agitated, complaining of palpitations. On auscultation there is good air movement, but the recovery room nurse notices an irregular heartbeat.

Expected actions:

1. Call for help
2. Provide supplemental oxygen
3. Evaluate the EKG and other vital signs.

Scenario continued:

With some help, a nasal cannula is placed with 2 l/min flow of oxygen. In his agitation, the patient has taken off some of the EKG leads. His HR per pulse oximeter is 189, BP 90/65, oxygen saturation 91%. Suddenly, the patient loses consciousness.

Expected actions:

1. Call for the crash cart
2. Assess the patient via circulation, airway, breathing
3. Follow the ACLS tachycardia
4. Reattach the EKG leads and assess the EKG
5. Increase IV fluids
6. Place mask with 6 l/min oxygen assuming spontaneous ventilation is present or start bag mask ventilation in the absence of such
7. Retake the vital signs.

Scenario continued:

The patient is breathing with a patent airway; a pulse, though very rapid is palpable, but irregular; the EKG shows a polymorphic ventricular tachycardia with twisting of QRS complexes. The vitals are HR 187, BP 89/63, SpO_2 96% with oxygen mask.

Expected actions:

1. Identify torsades de pointes
2. Prepare and administer magnesium IV
3. Attach the defibrillator.

Scenario continued:

While the magnesium is being administered, the rhythm shown on the defibrillator monitor changes to ventricular fibrillation.

Expected actions:

1. Follow the ACLS algorithm for pulseless cardiac arrest
   - Defibrillate immediately
   - CPR
   - Repeat defibrillation if shockable rhythm persists
   - CPR: consider advanced airway and epinephrine.

Scenario continued:

After two defibrillations the rhythm changes to sinus bradycardia. The patient resumes spontaneous ventilation.

Expected actions:

1. Follow the ACLS algorithm for post-arrest care
2. Assess patient including vital signs
3. Continue to monitor patient for recurrent torsades de pointes or ventricular fibrillation
4. After patient is stabilized, prepare the patient for transportation to an acute care hospital.

Scenario continued:

The drill ends with the patient regaining consciousness and being transported, with a physician, via ambulance to the nearest acute care hospital.

Debriefing

A debriefing, especially if drills did not go as well as hoped for, is difficult to do. It requires practice to give good feedback to correct misinformation, but also acknowledgment that different approaches are possible and no clear superior approach is identifiable. It is advisable to work with a partner to enable both to help each other improve their debriefing skills.

The following questions should guide the debriefing:

1. Identify three or more things the team felt went well with the scenario.
2. Identify three or more things the team felt they should have done differently.
3. What equipment was difficult to locate or use?
4. Was a clear leader directing the interventions?
5. Was there input from all team members and was it appropriately acknowledged?
6. Was there clear communication, and if not how can it be improved?
7. Were cognitive aids asked for and used? If not, how can this be encouraged?

8. Were the underlying problems identified early and addressed appropriately?
9. Did the team react quickly to changes in the scenario?
10. Which processes worked and which did not?
11. What strategies can be implemented to improve how these scenarios or similar situations are addressed in the future?

Discussion

The PACU is designed for observation of patients during a time when they are especially vulnerable to complications. Although the overall incidence of complications in the PACU, according to a study presented at the 2013 American Society of Anesthesiologists (ASA) Annual Meeting, decreased by nearly 60% between 1990 and 2010, it is still 9.9%[1]. The most common postoperative complications are nausea and vomiting (5.5%), hypotension (1.5%), upper airway obstruction (1.0%), hypertension (0.9%), dysrhythmias (0.5%), and major cardiac events (0.5%). Other complications include disorientation, persistent somnolence, hyper- or hypothermia, cerebrovascular accidents, peripheral nerve deficits, drug reactions, sore throat, and ocular complaints. The likelihood of any of these complications to occur depends on the patient population, procedure for which the patient presented, comorbidities, and the anesthetic. A thorough preoperative evaluation and careful planning of the anesthetic management and postoperative patient disposition can prevent a large percentage of complications.

The timely recognition of potentially life-threatening postoperative complications and the preparedness of all members of the healthcare team in the PACU is essential for a successful outcome. Part of being prepared is the availability of necessary equipment and medications for treatment, but more important is adequate training of providers. Being well versed in advanced cardiac life support, be it for the pediatric or adult patient, as well as regular refreshers in the form of drills, can improve patient outcome.[2]

Scenario 1: Postoperative upper airway obstruction

The incidence of postoperative upper airway obstruction is, as mentioned, approximately 1% and as such the third most commonly encountered complication in the PACU.[1] Left untreated it can lead to oxygen desaturation, hypoxia, and cardiac arrest. A systematic approach to the assessment and treatment can be helpful in addressing this potential life-threatening situation (Figure 5. 1).

The signs of upper airway obstruction include decreased or absent air movement, retractions (intercostal, substernal), and paradoxical breathing (opposite movement of abdomen and chest during inspiration). An upper airway obstruction can be complete, and therefore silent, or partial accompanied by either snoring (supra-laryngeal obstruction) or inspiratory stridor (peri-laryngeal obstruction). A common cause for upper airway obstruction is obstructive sleep apnea (OSA), which is more prevalent in the obese population and often undiagnosed.[3] Another risk group are patients following adeno-tonsillectomy for adeno-tonsillar hypertrophy, in which the risk for postoperative upper airway obstruction persists in up to 45%.[4]

In our case the patient had significant risk factors for postoperative upper airway obstruction. He suffered from a complete airway obstruction, as indicated by the silent respiratory effort and lack of air movement. The most likely etiology under these circumstances is soft tissue collapse and incomplete recovery from anesthesia, with decreased strength and coordination of the intrinsic and extrinsic airway muscles. The latter causes the tongue to fall back and obstruct the airway. Recommendation for initial treatment involves administration of 100% oxygen, chin lift/jaw thrust, and/or continuous positive airway pressure (CPAP), which often is sufficient to relieve the obstruction. In cases where it is not, insertion of an oral or nasal airway is indicated. Caution must be exercised when attempting to insert an oral airway. This should only be done in the unconscious patient, since it can otherwise trigger a significant gag reflex and vomiting. When placing a nasal airway, care must be exercised not to cause bleeding. The surgeon and/or anesthesiologist should be present. In addition, positioning the patient in the lateral decubitus or even prone position can help relieve the airway obstruction.[5] This can be challenging in the obese population.

Once the upper airway obstruction has been relieved the cause should be identified. In our scenario one has to consider residual pharmacological effects such as residual inhalational or intravenous anesthetics, prolonged neuromuscular blockade, narcotics, and benzodiazepines, to name a few. The decision to observe or reverse the effects of the medication needs to be based on the presenting situation.

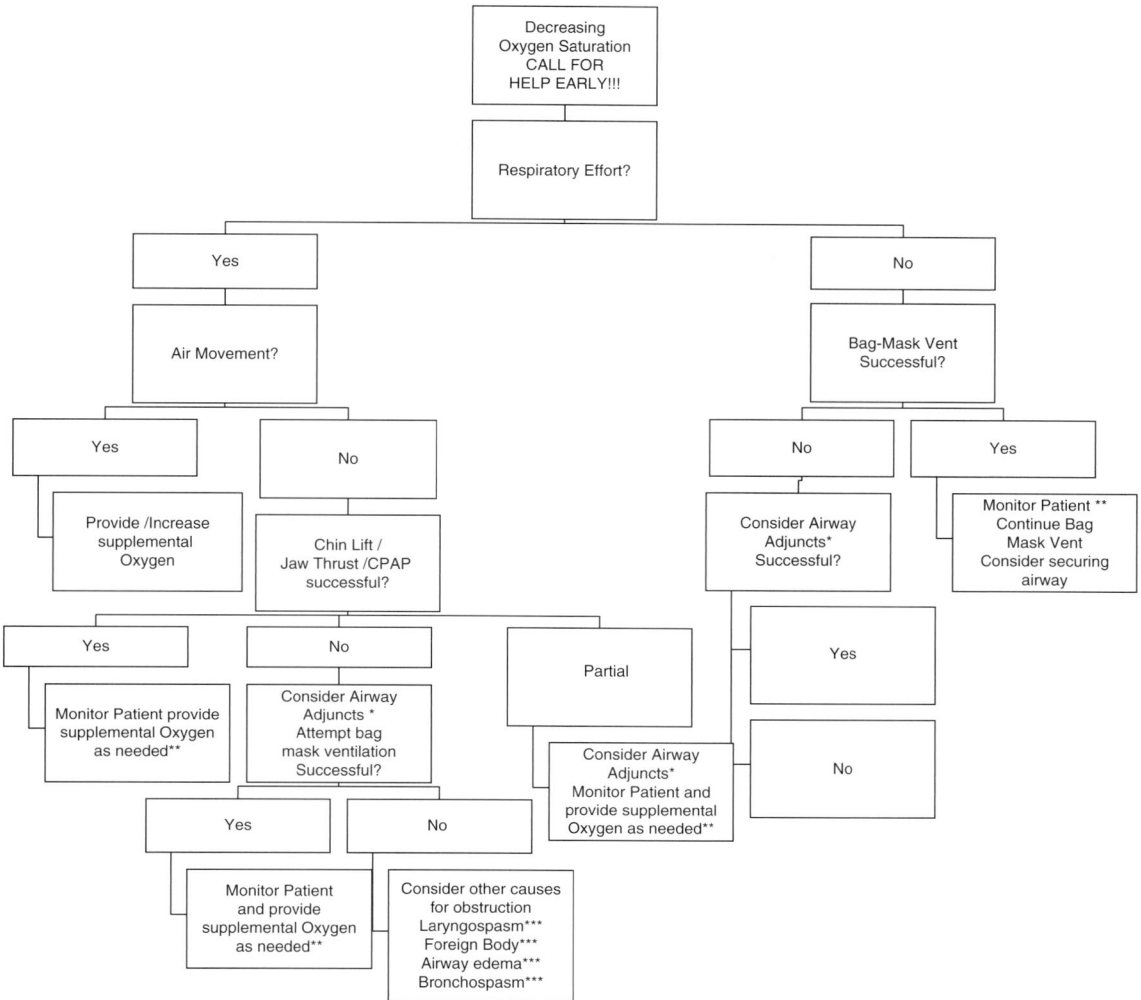

Figure 5.1 Airway Obstruction Algorithm

* Nasal or oral airway. *Cave*: Do not insert oral airway in awake or semiconscious patient

** Try to identify the cause for the obstruction and treat accordingly

*** See text for further interventions

The differential diagnosis in cases of complete or partial airway obstruction in the postoperative period has to include laryngospasm. It was excluded in our case by the ability to mask ventilate. Secretions or a foreign body in the glottis may cause laryngospasm during emergence. This involves violent contraction of the vocal cords impairing spontaneous air movement as well as bag ventilation. There are two different mechanisms involved eliciting different symptoms and requiring different treatments. Inspiratory stridor signifies loss of tone of the laryngeal abductor muscles. Complete cessation of airflow indicates a ball valve obstruction that occurs at the level of the true vocal cords, the false vocal cords, and the redundant supraglottic tissue. The first of these can be treated by removal of irritants (suctioning of secretions – *cave*: may trigger complete obstruction), jaw thrust, and positive pressure ventilation (PPV). The latter is treated by jaw thrust only, since PPV worsens the obstruction.[6] Should there be no improvement with the respective measures, propofol and/or succinylcholine with possible intubation is warranted.

A foreign body in the airway can also lead to a complete airway obstruction unlikely to be relieved by PPV, jaw thrust, or propofol/succinylcholine. This would require a direct laryngoscopy and removal of the foreign body.

Table 5.1 Differential diagnosis of perioperative non-febrile hyperthermia (not comprehensive)

Passive hyperthermia (warming devices)

Thyrotoxicosis or thyroid storm

Malignant hyperthermia

Neuroleptic malignant syndrome

Anticholinergic effect

Another potential differential diagnosis in the described scenario is airway edema. This can be caused by airway manipulation (i.e. intubation), allergic reaction, or under other circumstances such as the administration of large volumes of fluid, head neck surgery, or prolonged prone position. The treatment includes 100% oxygen, head elevation, fluid restriction, racemic epinephrine (*cave*: requires prolonged observation of patient, >2 h), dexamethasone, and/or reintubation.

Patients that underwent different surgical procedures may present with upper airway obstruction of a different etiology – for example, external compression of the airway secondary to hematoma or tight dressings after neck surgery, which may require relief via opening of sutures or removal of dressings.

This illustrates the need for evaluation and treatment of upper airway obstructions in the PACU in the context of the medical history, surgical procedure, anesthetic, and presentation.

Scenario 2: Hyperthermia in recovery room

The normal body temperature taken orally is 36.8 ± 0.5°C depending on the time of day.[7] It is regulated by a negative feedback system in the hypothalamus and maintained within a few tenths of 1°C by increases in heat production (thermogenesis)/heat loss (vasodilation/sweating) or decreases in heat loss (vasoconstriction).

Hypothermia is the most common temperature disturbance in the perioperative period. Nevertheless, hyperthermia is in all likelihood more dangerous than a comparable degree of hypothermia, especially if it is of a magnitude more than a few degrees Celsius.[8] When encountering elevations in body temperature, it is important to distinguish between febrile and non-febrile hyperthermia. Febrile hyperthermia is caused by an increase in the thermoregulatory set point secondary to either exogenous pyrogens or the release of endogenous pyrogens, such as in cases of infection, deep

venous thrombosis, or cancer.[9] Non-febrile hyperthermia is an increase of body temperature above the thermoregulatory set point. The differential diagnosis ranges from benign causes to life-threatening disease processes (Table 5.1).

Independent of the etiology, the elevation of body temperature can lead to significant morbidity in the susceptible patient. Hyperthermia causes an increase in metabolic rate, heart rate, respiratory rate, and oxygen consumption and possible acidosis. Patients suffering from coronary artery disease may develop cardiac ischemia. Compensatory mechanisms, e.g. sweating, vasodilatation, can lead to hypotension and dehydration. Specific disease processes or drug reactions can be fatal if left untreated. Therefore the treatment of hyperthermia must address the underlying cause and should not be aimed only at decreasing body temperature. If the anesthetic involved the use of triggering agents (as in our scenario), malignant hyperthermia (MH) treatment should be initiated until MH can be excluded. The treatment of MH is addressed in Chapter 3.

Non-febrile hyperthermia tends to improve with active patient cooling, unlike febrile hyperthermia, where it may fail to reduce body temperature and instead aggravate the situation by causing discomfort, shivering, and autonomic nervous system activation.[8] Cooling should be considered when the body temperature exceeds 39°C. In milder cases, removing covers and lowering the ambient temperature may be sufficient. Severe cases may require ice application, cooled IV fluids, or more invasive measures.[10]

In our scenario the underlying cause for the hyperthermia was thyroid storm or decompensated thyrotoxicosis (excess thyroid hormone), which can be precipitated by surgical stress in the un- or inadequately treated hyperthyroid patient and may present intraoperatively or up to 18 h postoperatively.[11] It is potentially life threatening and presents with some or all of the following: hyperthermia, severe tachycardia, atrial fibrillation, hypertension or hypotension (the latter secondary to cardiac decompensation or dehydration), myocardial ischemia, congestive heart failure, nausea and vomiting, diarrhea and seizures. The treatment can be divided into supportive therapy (fluids, cooling, acetaminophen); blocking of adrenergic-like effects (including rate control of atrial fibrillation [beta-blocker, i.e. esmolol, propranolol, or diltiazem]); reduction of T_3–T_4 conversion (hydrocortisone 100 mg IV every 8 h); and blocking of thyroid

Table 5.2 Key symptoms of anticholinergic syndrome

Pupillary dilation
Vasodilation/flushing
Hyperthermia
Dry skin
Hallucinations/agitation
Ileus/urinary retention
Tachycardia

hormone production and release.[12] In case of seizures, treatment with lorazepam is recommended.[13]

The most benign differential in this case scenario would be overheating via a warming device. The case lasted much longer than anticipated and a forced air heating device can lead to hyperthermia, which should improve with removal of covers and observation.

Additionally, the patient received glycopyrrolate, an anticholinergic medication that blocks the effects of acetylcholine in the central and peripheral nervous systems. Other medications in this class include atropine and scopolamine. These can all cause symptoms of an anticholinergic syndrome (Table 5.2) to varying degrees.

The effects of anticholinergic medications are completely reversible and will diminish as the causative agent is excreted and only supportive treatment is needed. In extreme, potentially life-threatening cases, physostigmine, a parasympathomimetic alkaloid and cholinesterase inhibitor, can be administered with caution.[14]

Lastly, neuroleptic malignant syndrome can exhibit a symptomatology similar to malignant hyperthermia; thyrotoxicosis and anticholinergic syndrome characterized by hyperthermia; generalized hypertonicity of skeletal muscles; elevated creatinine phosphokinase; instability of the autonomic nervous system (labile blood pressure, tachycardia, cardiac dysrhythmias); and altered mental status. It is associated with the use of neuroleptic medications (e.g. risperidone, haloperidol, prochlorperazine), abrupt discontinuation of neuroleptic medications or levodopa in patients with Parkinson's disease, or the use of dopamine-depleting agents. It is potentially fatal if not recognized early and treated appropriately. The treatment involves cessation of all neuroleptic medications and mainly supportive therapy (cooling, hydration, cardiovascular support). Secondary complications (hypoxia, acidosis, renal

failure) need to be treated aggressively to ensure a positive outcome.[15]

Scenario 3: Postoperative dysrhythmia

The overall incidence of perioperative dysrhythmias is 0.5% according to a study by Dabu-Bondor.[1] These are commonly found after cardiac or major non-cardiac surgery, but they can also be encountered in the ambulatory care setting. Predisposing factors and possible etiologies include increased sympathetic outflow secondary to hypercapnia, pain, agitation or hypoxia; electrolyte and acid base imbalances; preexisting cardiac conditions; myocardial ischemia; advanced age; medications; thyrotoxicosis; and malignant hyperthermia.[16] Identification of the underlying cause is a prerequisite for the treatment of dysrhythmias in the recovery room. Most of the time, medical treatment of the rhythm disturbance will suffice. In the presence of hemodynamic instability or deterioration to a malignant tachyarrhythmia, cardioversion or defibrillation, respectively, may be required. See Table 5.3 for a list of dysrhythmias and possible treatments. Following the Advanced Cardiac Life Support Guidelines of the American Heart Association[17] is strongly recommended.

New-onset atrial fibrillation is usually associated with cardiac or pulmonary surgery. In select cases it can be caused by metabolic imbalances such as thyrotoxicosis (see above). Treatment is aimed at rate control and the underlying cause.

The most common ventricular arrhythmias are isolated premature ventricular contractions (PVCs) and ventricular bigeminy. Neither is likely to deteriorate into life-threatening rhythms and usually do not require any treatment. Sinus tachycardia is also frequently encountered, resulting from increased sympathetic outflow, hyperthermia, congestive heart failure, or pulmonary embolus. Treatment should ensue after identification of the underlying cause. It does have the potential to cause increased morbidity in the susceptible patient by leading to myocardial ischemia secondary to increased oxygen consumption and decreased oxygen supply, in which case pharmacological rate control with either a beta-blocker or ditiazem even prior to identification of the underlying cause is advised.

Sinus bradycardia can be the result of opioid administration with the exception of meperidine, a high neuroaxial block, vagal stimulation, or beta-blockade

Table 5.3 Select postoperative dysrhythmias and treatment suggestions

Dysrhythmia	Treatment*

New-onset atrial fibrillation	Treat underlying cause
	Rate control:
	    Pharmacological if hemodynamically stable (beta-blocker or diltiazem)
	    Synchronized cardioversion if unstable

Premature ventricular contractions and bigeminy	Usually not required unless multifocal/ Reversible, which should be identified and addressed
Sinus tachycardia	Treat underlying cause Rate control if patient at risk for myocardial ischemia or heart failure
Sinus bradycardia	Treat underlying cause Administer atropine if symptomatic (hypotensive, disoriented, complaining of chest discomfort, in heart failure or shock) Consider pacing, dopamine or epinephrine infusion if ineffective[17]
Tachyarrhythmia (with pulse)	Treat underlying cause Consider sedated synchronized cardioversion if symptomatic (hypotensive, disoriented, complaining of chest discomfort, in heart failure or shock) If narrow QRS and stable, consider vagal maneuvers, adenosine, beta-blockers or calcium channel blockers If wide QRS and stable, consider adenosine (if regular and monomorphic), antiarrhythmic infusion[17]
Tachyarrhythmias (without pulse)	Defibrillation and resuscitation according to ACLS guidelines
Torsades de pointes	Magnesium infusion Beta-1 agonist for acquired QT prolongation (*Contraindicated in congenital QT prolongation*) Transcutaneous pacing Defibrillation in case of deterioration to ventricular fibrillation

* Monitor BP and SpO$_2$ closely; obtain ECG for rhythm diagnosis if possible and do not delay treatment; administer O$_2$ and provide assistant ventilation if necessary.

and only requires treatment if the patient develops symptoms of hypoperfusion (altered mental status, myocardial ischemia, shock, heart failure).

Sustained ventricular tachyarrhythmias are unusual in patients with a structurally normal heart and no cardiac history. Most commonly a history of coronary artery disease with an acute ischemic event or a healed myocardial infarction can be elicited. However, as mentioned previously, physiologic stress and metabolic imbalances can precipitate their occurrence. Idiopathic left ventricular tachycardia and idiopathic ventricular fibrillation are potentially lethal tachyarrhythmias that may occur in healthy individuals.[18] Identification and treatment of the underlying cause should be the goal, unless the patient is hemodynamically unstable or suffering from a lethal arrhythmia, in which cases either direct current cardioversion in

dysrhythmias amenable to such intervention or defibrillation is indicated.

Perioperative torsades de pointes, the arrhythmia in our scenario, is a rare polymorphic ventricular tachycardia with a distinctive ECG pattern of gradually changing amplitude and twisting of the QRS complex. It is seen in patients with either congenital or acquired QT prolongation, bradycardia, and electrolyte imbalances, such as hypokalemia, hypomagnesemia, and hypocalcemia and can be precipitated by catecholamine release. Diuretics and proton pump inhibitors can cause these imbalances. The timing for the occurrence of torsades is mainly intra- and postoperatively and medications implicated in worsening or causing the precipitating QT prolongation include, among others, sevoflurane, dolasetron, erythromycin, and ciprofloxacin.[19] The HR in torsades de pointes can range from 160 to 240 beats per minute. It often is self-limited, but can cause palpitations and syncope, as well as degenerate into ventricular fibrillation.[20] The treatment involves magnesium infusion (1–2 g over 30–60 s; can be repeated after 5–15 min) followed by close monitoring for potential side effects such as muscular weakness and beta-1 adrenergic agonists (*only* in cases of acquired QT prolongation, *contraindicated* in congenital QT prolongation). Patients with congenital QT prolongation benefit from beta-blockers because of a suspected underlying abnormal sympathetic tone. Transvenous pacing is an option for both patient groups. DC cardioversion should be a last resort because of the paroxysmal nature of torsades de pointes and the high recurrence rate after cardioversion. Defibrillation is needed should it deteriorate to ventricular fibrillation.[21]

In any case, if postoperative arrhythmias requiring intervention, be they pharmacological or electrical, occur the patient needs to be closely monitored and should be transferred to an acute care hospital for further evaluation and treatment.

References

1. S. M. Dabu-Bondoc, R. Hines, K. Shelley, et al. Complications in the Postanesthesia Care Unit: Then and Beyond. Presented at the ASA Annual Meeting 2013.
2. L. Knigh, et al. Improving code team performance and survival outcomes: Implementation of pediatric resuscitation team training. *Crit Care Med* 2014; 42: 243–251.
3. T. Young, M. Palta, J. Dempsey, et al. The occurence of sleep disordered breathing among middle aged adults. *N Engl J Med* 1993;328:1230–1235.
4. S. R. Shott. Evaluation and management of pediatric obstructive sleep apnea beyond tonsillectomy and adenoidectomy. *Current Opinions in Otolaryngology & Head and Neck Surgery* 2011; 19: 449–454.
5. Practice guidelines for the perioperative management of patients with obstructive sleep apnea. *Anesthesiology* 2014;120: 268–286.
6. M. Ramez Salem, G. J. Crystal, U. Nimmagadda. Understanding the mechanism of laryngospasm is crucial for proper treatment. *Anesthesiology* 2012; 117: 441–442.
7. P. A. Mackowiak, S. S. Wasserman, M. M. Levine. A critical appraisal of 98.6 degree F, the upper limit of the normal body temperature, and other legacies of Carl Reinhold August Wunderlich. *JAMA* 1992; 268; 12: 1578–1580.
8. D. I. Sessler. Chapter 54: Temperature regulation and monitoring. *Miller's Anesthesia* 2015: 1622–1646.
9. J. Stitt. Chapter 59: Regulation of body temperature. *Medical Physiology: A Cellular And Molecular Approach* 2003. 130.
10. M.M. Vu. Chapter 101: Hyperthermia. *Complications in Anesthesia* 2007:423–425.
11. A. P. Reed. Case 27: Thyroid disease. *Clinical Cases in Anesthesia* 2014:129–133.
12. J. Klubo-Gwiezdzinska, L. Wartofsky. Thyroid emergencies. *Medical Clinics of North America* 2012; 96; 2: 385–403.
13. D. Treiman, P. Meyers, N. Walton, et al. A comparison of four treatments for generalized convulsive status epilepticus. *New Engl J Med* 1998; 339: 792–798.
14. L. Culpepper, J. A. Lieberman, III. Correction. *Prim Care Companion CNS Disord* 2012; 14: 1: PCC.12lcx01326
15. P. Adnet, P. Lestavel, R. Krivostic-Horber. Neuroleptic malignant syndrome. *Br J Anaesth* 2000;85; 1: 129–135.
16. D. Driconsescu, L. Grecu. The postanesthesia care unit. *Clinical Anesthesia Procedures of the Massachusetts General Hospital.* 2007: 626.
17. 2010 American Heart Association Guidelines for Cardiopulmonary Resuscitation and Emergency Cardiovascular Care. *Circulation* 2010;122,18 suppl. 3.
18. J. L. Atlee. Chapter 79: Perioperative tachyarrhythmias. *Complications in Anesthesia* 2007: 319–323.
19. J. Johnston, S. Pal, P. Nagele. Perioperative torsade de pointes: A systematic review of published case reports. *Anesth Analg* 2013;117: 559–564.
20. AHA/ACCF Scientific Statement: Prevention of torsade de pointes in hospital settings. *Circulation* 2010;121: 1047–1060.
21. J. Dave, J. N. Rottman, et al. Torsade de Pointes. 9/2014. Medscape article 1950863

Chapter

6

Acute pulmonary embolism

Shyamal Asher and David M. Dickerson

Introduction

Pulmonary embolism, a potential complication of surgical and medical hospitalization, is a leading cause of morbidity and mortality. One study of over seven million patients found postoperative venous thromboembolism (VTE) to be the second most common medical complication and cause of extended hospital stay.[1] As ambulatory surgical centers take on more complex surgical procedures and higher-risk patients, the potential for thromboembolic events in this setting will also increase. In a recent study of surgical outcomes using a multi-center database study, the 30-day incidence of VTE for outpatient surgery was 1.18% among high-risk patients.[2] This chapter aims to provide a guide for patient risk stratification, the methods for diagnosis, and the treatment of embolic events in the ambulatory center.

Scenario 1: Embolism in the operating room

Following a fall, a 54-year-old male is undergoing internal fixation of a tibial plateau fracture under general anesthesia. After release of the tourniquet, the patient's oxygen saturations drop from 99 to 85% on 40% FiO_2 and heart rate increases from 75 to 110 with a stable blood pressure.

Expected actions:

1. Notify surgical team of acute changes while ruling out other causes of desaturation and tachycardia
2. Increase FiO_2
3. Monitor blood pressure.

Scenario continued:

Fraction inspired oxygen is increased to 100% with improvement in oxygen saturation. The end-tidal CO_2 is noted to decrease from 38 to 25. Blood pressure has fallen to the low limits of normal.

Expected actions:

1. Communicate changes to surgeon, call for help
2. Check arterial blood gas (ABG), consider arterial line for serial sampling of arterial oxygen levels and for hemodynamic monitoring
3. Recognize signs and symptoms of pulmonary embolism including calculation of A-a gradient.

Scenario continued:

An ABG is drawn and found to be pH 7.25, PO_2 85, bicarbonate 26, and O_2 sat 95% on 100% FiO_2. Blood pressure remains stable, but at the low limits of normal.

Expected actions:

1. Perform echocardiography, if available.

Scenario continued:

Arterial blood gases continue to show hypoxia with large oxygen gradient and high clinical suspicion for pulmonary embolism. Surgeon suggests heparinization. No echocardiography available. Patient exhibits persistent hypoxia despite increased FiO_2.

Expected actions:

1. Ensure adequate oxygenation and circulation
2. Consider anticoagulation after discussion with surgeon. Assuming no heparin allergy, administer 5000 units heparin IV with infusion of 18 units/kg/h checking partial thromboplastin time (ptt). If massive embolism expected, consider 10,000 units heparin IV with 1500 units/h
3. Monitor hemoglobin and for signs of surgical bleeding. Rule out stigmata of fat embolism syndrome, specifically, a petechial rash

Perioperative Drill-Based Crisis Management, ed. Steven Butz. Published by Cambridge University Press. © Cambridge University Press 2016.

4. Contact nearest medical center for transfer, admission, and further diagnostic testing and possible thrombectomy.

Scenario continued:

Drill ends with arrangements for transfer.

Scenario 2: Embolism in recovery room (or medical unit)

You receive a page from the recovery room nurse that a 72-year-old female status post laparoscopic right hemicolectomy for colonic adenocarcinoma is experiencing shortness of breath. She had an uneventful, general endotracheal anesthetic and had no issues on sign-out to recovery nursing 15 minutes prior.

Expected actions:

1. Evaluate the patient with focus on vital signs, mental status and perform focused cardiac and pulmonary exam.

Scenario continued:

The patient is awake and talking, complaining of worsening shortness of breath. Her oxygen requirement is increased. She is receiving 50% oxygen by facemask with an oxygen saturation of 90%. Her vitals are BP 100/60, pulse 115, respiratory rate 30.

She appears to have increased work of breathing. Lungs are clear to auscultation bilaterally.

Expected actions:

1. Notify surgical team of change in patient's status while ruling out alternative causes of hypoxemia in the PACU, including excessive opioid administration and residual neuromuscular blockade. Ensure oxygen is being delivered
2. Consider securing her airway and ordering additional diagnostic testing such as chest x-ray and arterial blood gas.

Scenario continued:

The patient suddenly deteriorates with worsening mental status, worsening respiratory distress with oxygen saturation now in mid 80s, and hypotension with mean arterial pressures in the 40s. This is rapidly followed by ventricular fibrillation.

Expected actions:

1. Call for help
2. Follow Advanced Cardiac Life Support Guidelines:
   a. Defibrillate immediately
   b. CPR
   c. Secure airway, consider epinephrine and vasopressin as per ACLS algorithm
   d. Check ABG; consider arterial line, central access.

Scenario continued:

Return of spontaneous circulation is achieved after 10 min of ACLS and two rounds of epinephrine. Patient is now intubated and with a BP at the low limit of normal.

Blood gas shows a large A-a and CO_2 gradient. An ECG shows an $S_1Q_3T_3$ pattern. Pulmonary embolism is highly suspected.

Expected actions:

1. Consider echocardiography and other diagnostic testing to diagnose pulmonary embolism, consider CT scan, and activate pulmonary embolism protocol if available
2. If high suspicion for pulmonary embolism and assuming no contraindication, anticoagulate with heparin
3. Contact nearest medical center for transfer, admission, and further diagnostic testing, and possible thrombectomy.

Scenario continued:

Drill ends with arrangements for transfer.

Scenario 3: Fat embolism in the operating room

A 65-year-old female is undergoing open reduction internal fixation (ORIF) with an intramedullary nail for a left femur fracture under epidural anesthesia with sedation. Soon after nail insertion, the patient suddenly becomes restless, tachypneic to the mid 30s, with decreasing oxygen saturation.[18]

Expected actions:

1. Notify surgical team of acute changes while ruling out other causes of tachypnea and desaturation and restlessness including aspiration,

Table 6.1 Identifying patients at risk for venous thromboembolism (VTE)

Patient Factors	Surgery Factors	Anesthesia/Medical Factors
• Fracture of pelvis, hip, or long bones • Multiple trauma • Malignancy • Prior VTE • Age[2] >40 • Obesity[2] – BMI >40 • Immobility • Inflammatory disorders such as IBD[5]	• Major general surgery – abdominal or thoracic • Orthopedic surgery including arthroscopic surgery • Venous surgery – at saphenofemoral junction and non-great saphenous vein surgery[2]	• Failure to administer prophylaxis • Time under general anesthesia

Abbreviations used: BMI – Body Mass Index; IBD – inflammatory bowel disease; VTE – venous thromboembolism.

excessive epidural blockade, pain, or stage 2 consciousness-associated disinhibition

2. Call for help
3. Notify surgical team of acute changes
4. Assess sedation level compared to immediately prior, check for conjugate gaze, assist patient ventilation with mask, rule out aspiration.

Scenario continued:

Oxygen saturation has decreased to the mid 80s. Ventricular bigeminy noted on ECG. The restlessness rapidly progresses to a generalized seizure.

Expected actions:

1. Consider giving seizure abortive therapy such as a benzodiazepine if seizure persists
2. Intubate the patient once it is safe to manipulate the airway.

Scenario continued:

Within seconds, the oxygen saturation cannot be recorded and no pulse can be palpated.

Expected actions:

1. Notify surgical team and begin CPR
2. Follow Advanced Cardiac Life Support guidelines
   a. Defibrillate
   b. CPR
   c. Consider epinephrine and vasopressin as per ACLS algorithm.
   d. Ensure adequate venous access, consider arterial line.

Scenario continued:

Return of spontaneous circulation is achieved. Patient is now intubated and with a blood pressure at the low limit of normal.

Expected actions:

1. Consider chest radiograph, echocardiography and other diagnostic testing such as ABG sampling
2. Examine skin and mucous membranes for a petechial rash that would suggest a fat embolism. If no rash, low likelihood of fat embolism. Consider other causes of hemodynamic instability including myocardial infarction, pneumothorax, or venous thromboembolism due to deep vein thrombus
4. Continue supportive management, maintaining perfusion and oxygenation. If high suspicion for pulmonary embolism and assuming no contraindication, anticoagulate with heparin
3. Contact nearest medical center for transfer, admission, and further diagnostic testing.

Scenario continued:

Drill ends with arrangements for transfer.

Discussion

Identifying at-risk patients

Specific patient, surgical, and medical factors contribute to VTE risk (Table 6.1). Provider recognition of risk factors may heighten suspicion for pulmonary embolism (PE), improving time to diagnosis and treatment. Furthermore, the identification of risk factors for PE or VTE, and the potential subsequent recognition of a deep vein thrombus preoperatively, may prompt

Table 6.2 Characterizing non-thrombotic embolic events[6]

Embolism Contents	Mechanism	Clinical characteristics
Fat	Classically, after pelvic or long bone fractures due to release of fat into systemic circulation from the bone marrow; may also occur with placement of an intramedullary rod	Fat embolism syndrome: hypoxia, respiratory distress, mental status changes, petechial rash on anterior surface of neck, thorax, and mucous membranes
Carbon dioxide	Insufflation gas via trocar or needle inadvertently placed IV during laparoscopy	Hypoxia, dyspnea, acute drop in $ETCO_2$ or $PaCO_2$, tachypnea, tachycardia, hypotension
Air	Requires communication between source of air and vasculature and presence of gradient favoring intravascular entry of air, common during craniotomy, cesarean delivery, sitting position surgeries, central line placement or removal	Hypoxia, cough, dyspnea, acute drop in $ETCO_2$ or $PaCO_2$, tachypnea, hypotension
Amniotic fluid	Translocation of amniotic fluid into venous circulation acutely or within 24 h of delivery	Hypoxia, cough, dyspnea, acute drop in $ETCO_2$ or $PaCO_2$, tachypnea, hypotension, presence of fetal cells in central line aspirate, pulmonary edema, convulsions, coagulopathy

Abbreviations used: $ETCO_2$ – end tidal carbon dioxide concentration; $PaCO_2$ – partial pressure of arterial carbon dioxide.

preoperative treatment or placement of an inferior vena cava filter to reduce risk. The Caprini risk assessment tool incorporates 20 patient characteristics that contribute to VTE, providing risk stratification into low, moderate, high, and highest risk.[3,4] In the Caprini risk assessment, recent trauma, stroke, pelvis, hip or leg fracture, or major lower extremity arthroplasty carry the highest risk of VTE. Such scoring tools are relevant as adequate VTE prophylaxis is risk dependent and prophylaxis can range from elastic stockings, intermittent pneumatic compression, and low-dose unfractionated heparin to low-molecular weight heparin or factor Xa inhibitors.

Non-thrombotic events create similar pathophysiology and cardiopulmonary compromise. During central line placement and removal, cesarean delivery, sitting position surgeries, craniotomy, orthopedic procedures, and laparoscopy, vigilance is essential for early detection and treatment of these non-thrombotic embolic events. The characteristics and mechanisms of these events are listed in Table 6.2.

Diagnosis of acute pulmonary embolism

The clinical signs and symptoms of acute pulmonary embolism (PE), dyspnea, pleuritic chest pain, tachypnea, and tachycardia are non-specific as they are also common in patients without PE and are difficult to detect in patients under general anesthesia. A recent meta-analysis found empirical clinical assessment of PE to have a sensitivity of 85% but a specificity of 51%.[7] This result emphasizes the importance of additional diagnostic testing when acute PE is suspected. Tables 6.3 and 6.4 summarize the studies that may be performed and the expected result in the event of PE. Intraoperatively, the clinical picture may be less clear and marked solely by acute or gradual change in oxygen saturation or hemodynamics. The arterial blood gas and echocardiography may be the most readily available assessments while the other tests listed in Tables 6.3 and 6.4 may help delineate such a process in the recovery and monitoring phases of care.

Treatment of acute pulmonary embolism

The acute response requires prompt closed-loop communication and multidisciplinary care. Upon first suspicion of an embolic event, the anesthesia provider notifies the surgical and ancillary team and calls for help from other available anesthesia providers, depending on the patient's stability. After prompt communication with the surgical team, the surgeon

Table 6.3 Laboratory studies for pulmonary embolism

Study	Description/Finding	Data
Arterial blood gas	Usually reveals hypoxemia, hypocapnia, respiratory alkalosis, and an increased A-a gradient	Of limited value due to poor sensitivity[8]
Brain natriuretic peptide	A vasoactive hormone that is released from the cardiac ventricles in response to ventricular dilation	Low sensitivity and specificity[9]
Troponin increase	Present in 30–40% of patients who have PE. Thought to be secondary to acute right ventricular overload	Not useful for diagnosis but may be useful for prognosis[10]
D-dimer	A degradation product of cross-linked fibrin	Adequate sensitivity and negative predictive value

Abbreviations used: A-a gradient – alveolar to arterial gradient; ABG – arterial blood gas; PE– pulmonary embolism; RV – right ventricle.

Table 6.4 Imaging and studies in pulmonary embolism

Study	Findings	Data
EKG	Most commonly non-specific ST-segment and T-wave changes. Classic "$S_1Q_3T_3$" seen mostly with massive PE	Limited diagnostic usefulness[11]
CXR	Commonly include atelectasis, pleural effusion	Non-specific to PE, limited diagnostic usefulness[11]
Echocardiography	Right ventricular dilation and hypokinesis; septal flattening and paradoxical septal motion and direct visualization of pulmonary embolism;[12] small LV relative to RV with normal LV systolic function **McConnell's sign:** akinesia of the mid free wall, but normal apical motion (77% sensitive and 94% specific for PE)	Useful in rapid diagnosis to identify patients who may benefit from thrombolysis[13]
CT Angiography	Filling defects are seen in pulmonary veins after injection of IV contrast	Considered first line for diagnosis of PE. Sensitivity of 96–100%; specificity of 97–98%;[14] may be difficult to obtain intraoperatively or in an ambulatory surgical center

Abbreviations used: EKG – electrocardiogram; PE – pulmonary embolism; CXR – chest radiograph; LV – left ventricle; RV – right ventricle.

Table 6.5 Support and treatment for acute pulmonary embolism

Respiratory support	Consider intubation and mechanical ventilation for severe hypoxemia and respiratory failure
Hemodynamic support	IV fluids – limit to 500–1000 ml as excess fluid administration exacerbates RV failure Vasopressors – norepinephrine, dopamine, dobutamine are the preferred agents for PE-related shock[16]
Anticoagulation therapy	Should be administered to all patients with high or intermediate clinical probability of acute PE even without confirmatory imaging procedures; IV unfractionated heparin preferred[17]
Thrombolytic therapy	Indicated for patients with severe clinical manifestations including persistent shock due to acute PE
Surgical management	Includes catheter and surgical embolectomy; usual indication is systemic hypotension due to acute PE in a patient in whom thrombolysis has failed or is contraindicated
IVC filters	May be used for primary and secondary prevention

Abbreviations used: IV – intravenous; RV – right ventricle; PE – pulmonary embolism; IVC – inferior vena cava.

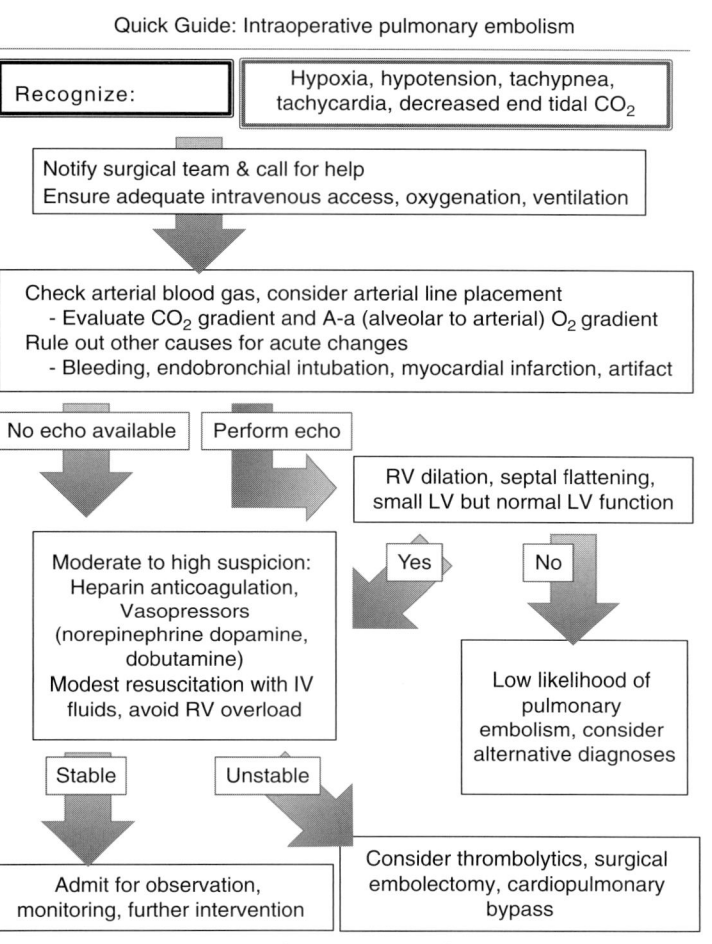

Quick Guide: Intraoperative pulmonary embolism

Recognize: Hypoxia, hypotension, tachypnea, tachycardia, decreased end tidal CO_2

Notify surgical team & call for help
Ensure adequate intravenous access, oxygenation, ventilation

Check arterial blood gas, consider arterial line placement
- Evaluate CO_2 gradient and A-a (alveolar to arterial) O_2 gradient
Rule out other causes for acute changes
- Bleeding, endobronchial intubation, myocardial infarction, artifact

No echo available

Perform echo

RV dilation, septal flattening, small LV but normal LV function

Moderate to high suspicion:
Heparin anticoagulation,
Vasopressors
(norepinephrine dopamine,
dobutamine)
Modest resuscitation with IV
fluids, avoid RV overload

Yes

No

Low likelihood of pulmonary embolism, consider alternative diagnoses

Stable

Unstable

Admit for observation, monitoring, further intervention

Consider thrombolytics, surgical embolectomy, cardiopulmonary bypass

Abbreviations: echo - echocardiography; LV - left ventricle;
RV - right ventricle; IV - intravenous

Figure 6.1 Quick guide for acute pulmonary embolism treatment

may minimize activity that worsens the embolism or affects the patient's hemodynamics. Adequate IV access should be obtained and an arterial catheter placed for continuous blood pressure monitoring and serial arterial blood sampling. If possible, echocardiography can help guide resuscitation and supportive therapy. The patient should be ventilated with 100% oxygen to minimize hypoxia-related PVR increases, and acidosis should be minimized through adequate minute ventilation and optimizing perfusion. Positive end expiratory pressure (PEEP) should be used cautiously as increased sustained transthoracic pressure may negatively impact venous return and cardiac output. Hypotension should be treated with IV fluids, with concern for right ventricular overload. Vasopressors with inotropic potential are preferred

to improve right ventricular function. Negative inotropes should be avoided. If the patient remains unstable and a thrombotic event is suspected, unfractionated heparin should be administered. Aspiration via a central venous catheter may relieve an air or CO_2 embolism. In the event the patient remains unstable or in a state of persistent cardiogenic shock, catheter or surgical embolectomy should be considered. Extracorporeal membrane oxygenation has been used for persistent cardiogenic shock despite rapid anticoagulation.[15]

In the ambulatory setting, supportive therapy and anticoagulation may be the most advanced and interventional treatment available and point-of-care echocardiography may not be available. Refractory conditions should be stabilized and the patient transferred for continued workup, monitoring, and potential intervention. If a patient's condition stabilizes, he or she should be monitored for signs or symptoms of recurrent embolism or thrombus extension until patient transfer to the nearest medical center. Severe cases may be accompanied by profound tachypnea and fatigue of the respiratory system necessitating continued mechanical ventilation. In the event of recovery, a suspicion for pulmonary embolism should result in hospital admission for continued monitoring, workup, and potential treatment.

Table 6.5 lists the support and treatment for acute pulmonary embolism, while Figure 6.1 summarizes a workflow that can serve as a guide for treatment or for conducting drills or simulations.

Conclusion

The catastrophic potential of embolic events in the ambulatory surgery center necessitates vigilance and preparedness by both anesthesiologist and the center. Heightened awareness, effective communication, and prompt diagnosis and treatment are necessary to optimize outcomes after acute pulmonary embolism.

References

1. Zhan C, Miller M. Excess length of stay, charges, and mortality attributable to medical injuries during hospitalization. *JAMA* 2003;290:1868–1874.
2. Pannucci CJ, Shanks A, Moote MJ, et al. Identifying patients at high risk for venous thromboembolism requiring treatment after outpatient surgery. *Ann Surg* 2012;255:1093–1099.
3. Caprini JA. Thrombosis risk assessment as a guide to quality patient care. *Dis Mon* 2005;51:70–78.
4. Bahl V, Hu HM, Henke PK, et al. A validation study of retrospective venous thromboembolism risk scoring method. *Ann Surg* 2010;251:344–350.
5. Zezos P, Kouklakis G, Saibil F, et al. Inflammatory bowel disease and thromboembolism. *World J Gastroenterol* 2014;20(38):13863–13878.
6. Jorens PG, Van Marck E, Snoeckx A, Parizel PM. Nonthrombotic pulmonary embolism. *Eur Respir J* 2009;452–474.
7. Lucassen W, Geersing GJ, Erkens PM, et al. Clinical decision rules for excluding pulmonary embolism: a meta-analysis. *Ann Intern Med* 2011;155:448–460.
8. Rodger MA, Carrier M, Jones GN, et al. Diagnostic value of arterial blood gas measurement in suspected pulmonary embolism. *Am J Respir Crit Care Med* 2000;162:2105–2108.
9. Sohne M, TenWolde M, Boomsma F, et al. Brain natriuretic peptide in hemodynamically stable pulmonary embolism. *J Thromb Haemost* 2006;4:552–556.
10. Meyer T, Binder L, Hruska N, et al. Cardiac troponin I elevation in acute pulmonary embolism is associated with right ventricular dysfunction. *J Am Coll Cardiol* 2000;36:1632–1636.
11. Stein PD, Saltzman HA, Weg JG, et al. Clinical characteristics of patients with acute pulmonary embolism. *Am J Cardiol* 1991;68:1723–1724.
12. Goldhaber S. Echocardiography in management of pulmonary embolism. *Ann Intern Med* 2002;136:691–700.
13. Mookadam F, Jiamsripong P, Goel R, et al. Critical appraisal on the utility of echocardiography in the management of acute pulmonary embolism. *Cardiol Rev* 2010;18:29–37.
14. Mos IC, Klok FA, Kroft LJ, et al. Imaging tests in the diagnosis of pulmonary embolism. *Semin Respir Crit Care Med* 2012;33:138–143.
15. Misawa Y, Fuse K, Yamaguchi T, et al. Mechanical circulatory assist for pulmonary embolism. *Perfusion* 2000; 15: 527–529
16. Kucher N, Goldhaber S. Management of massive pulmonary embolism. *Circulation* 2005;112:e28–e32.
17. Konstantinides S, Goldhaber S. Pulmonary embolism: risk assessment and management. *Eur Heart J* 2012;33:3014–3022.
18. Sarkar S, Mandal K, Bhattacharya P. Successful management of massive intraoperative pulmonary fat embolism with percutaneous cardiopulmonary support. *Indian J Crit Care Med* 2008;12(3):136–139.

Difficult airway

Connie K. Tran and Sonal N. Zambare

Introduction

Airway management in a lone-standing ambulatory surgical center has come under a lot of scrutiny after the death of a highly respected celebrity while undergoing an outpatient procedure from alleged complications related to loss of airway control. Airway management is fundamental to the practice of anesthesiology, whether care is provided at a lone standing ambulatory surgery care center, procedure room, or an operating room in a hospital. Inability to ventilate and oxygenate can lead to catastrophic outcomes. All anesthesia providers should be prepared to manage a difficult airway which may be easily predictable or may be encountered in an unanticipated scenario. The alternatives to provide adequate oxygenation when conventional methods have failed should be in every anesthesiologist's armamentarium. The anesthesia provider should have a careful plan for extubation for every patient since difficult airway and intubation can occur during this critical period. Every ambulatory center should have a guideline for hospital admission if needed and a portable difficult airway cart that is easily accessible.

The three scenarios presented below depict different situations where difficulty in ventilating, oxygenating, or intubating may be encountered. These cases emphasize that a thorough knowledge of the difficult airway algorithm and familiarity with the available airway equipment may prevent catastrophic outcomes.

Educational objectives

1. Be prepared to manage anticipated and unanticipated difficult airway
2. Develop strategies for extubation after encountering a difficult airway

3. Decide which patients need admission after a "scheduled" outpatient procedure.

Scenario 1: Pediatric difficult airway

A 4-year-old child, 16 kg, presents for a tonsillectomy and adenoidectomy.

He has Down's syndrome and a history of snoring. No cardiac abnormality is present. He has a small mouth, relatively large tongue, hypoplastic mandible, and short neck without atlanto-axial instability. No formal sleep study is available.

Expected actions:

1. Perform a comprehensive history and airway examination
2. Consider the possibility of central as well as obstructive sleep apnea
3. Anticipate difficulty in ventilation and intubation.

Scenario continued:

The anesthetic plan is for an inhalation induction followed by endotracheal intubation. The use of IV opioids and neuromuscular blocking agents is avoided. Multimodal analgesia is used with dexmedetomidine, IV acetaminophen.

On induction, there is severe airway obstruction and a drop in oxygen saturation.

Expected actions:

1. Apply jaw thrust and chin lift
2. Place an oral or nasopharyngeal airway
3. Use continuous positive airway pressure
4. Place an IV line quickly
5. Attempt to intubate quickly
6. Make sure ENT surgeon is immediately available.

Perioperative Drill-Based Crisis Management, ed. Steven Butz. Published by Cambridge University Press. © Cambridge University Press 2016.

Scenario continued:

An oropharyngeal airway was placed and mask ventilation was successful. A peripheral IV was placed easily. A direct laryngoscopy was attempted with a Miller 2 blade, but a grade 4 view was obtained. The attempt was aborted and mask ventilation commenced. Repeat attempt to intubate resulted in trauma to the tonsils and now there is profuse bleeding in the oral cavity. Mask ventilation is now difficult and oxygen saturation begins to drop to the 50s. HR is 30 bpm.

Expected actions:

1. Call for help
2. Call for code cart; activate code team
3. Call for difficult airway cart
4. Suction the oral cavity
5. Check pulse and if absent start chest compressions
6. Ask ENT surgeon to prepare to perform a cricothyroidotomy or tracheostomy.

Scenario continued:

Oral cavity is suctioned and while chest compressions are being performed; 1.6 ml of epinephrine 1:10,000 concentration given IV. Size 2 laryngeal mask airway (LMA) is placed in the oral cavity, and ventilation is possible via the LMA. Oxygen saturation improved to the low 90s, HR increasing to 100 bpm. Intubation is carried out using a fiberoptic bronchoscope via the LMA with size 4 ETT. Oxygen saturation is now 99% with normal BP and HR.

Expected actions:

1. Discussion with surgeon on the feasibility to proceed or defer surgery
2. A discussion with parents, surgeon, and anesthesia team ensued and because of the trauma to the tonsils with laryngoscopy attempts and the fact that the patient is now stable with good oxygen saturation and vital signs, a decision was made to proceed with surgery
3. Steroid given to reduce swelling
4. Anticipation of difficult emergence and extubation.

Scenario continued:

Surgery proceeded uneventfully. Patient was able to be extubated when widely awake. The child gets admitted for "23-hour observation" and is discharged the next day.

Scenario 2: Loss of natural airway during sedation

A 55-year-old man, 105 kg, 64 inches (162.5 cm) tall, BMI 40 kg/m^2 is in the GI suite for a colonoscopy for screening. He has a strong family history of colon cancer. He has a history of hypertension, well-controlled, type 2 diabetes, and severe reflux disease. His airway exam is Mallampatti class 3, with thyromental distance of 6 cm. He has a beard and a history of snoring. There is no formal sleep study performed.

The plan is to administer propofol and maintain spontaneous respirations, while providing supplemental oxygen via a nasal cannula. The patient is in right lateral position and total of 200 mg of propofol is given IV. The procedure is started. Shortly afterwards, the patient becomes apneic and saturations drop to 90%.

Expected actions:

1. Ensure use of capnography to rapidly detect apnea and hypoventilation
2. Rule out airway obstruction by placing an oral or a nasopharyngeal airway
3. Prepare to mask ventilate
4. Confirm the availability of difficult airway equipment including a video laryngoscope.

Scenario continued:

The end tidal carbon dioxide monitoring shows an apnea for about 30 s. Oral and nasopharyngeal airways placed. Mask ventilation is attempted; however it is difficult to achieve a tight seal with the face mask due to the beard. Pulse oximeter is now reading 80% and dropping rapidly.

Expected actions:

1. Call for help
2. Stop the procedure
3. Turn the patient to supine position
4. Attempt 2-hand mask ventilation.

Scenario continued:

It is still difficult to mask ventilate, even with assistance from another person. The oxygen saturation is now 60%.

Expected actions:

1. Call for difficult airway cart
2. Attempt to intubate with a video-assisted laryngoscope

3. Have supraglottic airway devices such as LMA for rescue
4. Consider emergency invasive airway access such as percutaneous cricothyroidotomy, jet ventilation, retrograde intubation.

Scenario continued:

Video laryngoscope arrived in the room and was used for intubation; a good view of the larynx and vocal cords is seen but difficulty is encountered in passing the ETT. Multiple attempts at passing the ETT through the vocal cords were unsuccessful and oxygen saturation now in the 50s. Decision made to abandon video-assisted laryngoscopy.

Size 5 LMA placed but unable to ventilate. Oxygen saturation now drops to the 30s.

Expected actions:

Anticipate emergency invasive airway:
1. Obtain cricothyroidotomy kit
2. Call for code team or emergency help
3. Check whether the general surgeon is available for possible surgical airway
4. Evaluate the need for CPR.

Scenario continued:

While waiting for the cricothyroidotomy kit to arrive, the anesthesiologist uses the videoscope and is able to place an Eschmann stylet through the vocal cords, then the ETT was railroaded over the stylet. The patient is successfully intubated and ventilated. Oxygen saturation recovers to 100%.

Expected actions:

1. Decision whether or not to resume procedure
2. Plan for possible difficult extubation
3. Plan for possible hospital admission
4. Document a careful note of difficult intubation, inform the patient and surgeon, and provide a difficult airway letter to patient and place a copy in the chart.

Scenario continued:

Since the patient is now well oxygenated and vital signs are stable, decision taken to resume procedure. The remainder of the case proceeds uneventfully. The patient is extubated when wide awake and breathing spontaneously and meets extubation criteria. The patient was then transported to the hospital for an overnight admission for monitoring.

Scenario 3: Unexpected difficult airway

A 50-year-old female is scheduled for an ORIF of the right ankle. Her medical history is significant for well-controlled, non-insulin-dependent diabetes mellitus (NIDDM) on metformin, arterial hypertension (HTN) on labetalol, gastroesophageal reflux disease (GERD), history of nighttime snoring, and BMI of 35. No surgical history, family history of anesthetic problems, or allergy to medications.

Physical exam shows a very nervous woman. Airway exam is significant for MP 2, mouth opening of two fingerbreadths, hyoid-mental of 5 cm, and neck has full range of motion.

The patient does not want any regional blocks because of "fear of needles" and wants general anesthesia only. She has been nil per os (NPO) for 10 h.

The plan is for GI prophylaxis with metoclopramide, famotidine, and citric acid/sodium citrate (non-particulate antacid) prior to induction and general endotracheal anesthesia (GETA) with direct laryngoscopy.

Mask ventilation is easy after induction, and 40 mg of rocuronium is given. Direct laryngoscopy with MAC 3 blade shows a Cormack–Lehane grade 4 view with a floppy epiglottis. You are unable to pass ETT. Second attempt after positioning shows a grade 3 view but still unable to pass ETT. Oxygen saturation begins to drop to low 90s.

Expected actions:

1. Begin masking with high-flow oxygen
2. Call for help
3. Call for difficult airway cart and video laryngoscope
4. Have a supraglottic device available.

Scenario continued:

Oxygen saturation continues to drop to low 80s and masking becomes more difficult. Oropharyngeal airway is placed. Mask ventilation is changed to two-hand ventilation while difficult airway cart is being located. Oxygen saturation rises to high 90s.

Expected actions:

1. Reassess
2. Proceed with alternative approach to intubation with alternative devices or different personnel.

Scenario continued:

An attempt with a Miller 2 blade is unsuccessful and ventilation is easy with two-hand technique. A size 4 laryngeal mask airway is placed but unable to ventilate via the airway device. Oxygen saturation decreases to the 80s. LMA is removed and patient is ventilated with two-hand face mask. Oxygen saturation returns to 99%.

Expected actions:

1. Reassess situation
2. Consider invasive airway access such as surgical or percutaneous airway, jet ventilation, or retrograde intubation
3. Consider feasibility of other options such as proceeding with surgery using facemask, laryngeal tube, or intubating LMA
4. Consider waking up the patient, re-preparation of the patient for an awake intubation, or cancelling surgery.

Scenario continued:

Intubation was successful by the second anesthesiologist using a size 4 intubating LMA and 7.0 ETT. Oxygen saturation 100% after suctioning ETT with small amount of blood-tinged secretion. Surgery proceeds uneventfully.

Expected actions:

1. Plan for extubation when patient is fully awake
2. Reversal of muscle relaxant given after nerve stimulator demonstrates full train of four (TOF)
3. Consider the placement of airway exchange catheter such as Aintree catheter or supraglottic device such as LMA prior to removal of ETT
4. Consider careful documentation of difficult intubation, informing the patient and surgeon, providing a difficult airway letter to patient and copy in the chart.

Scenario continued:

Patient is extubated at the end of procedure when fully awake, maintaining oxygenation and ventilation. A difficult airway letter is given to the patient, family member, and surgeon in the recovery room. A copy of the letter is placed in the patient chart. The patient may consider registering with a medical alert database company.

Debriefing

1. Identify up to three or more things the team felt went well with the scenario.
2. Identify up to three or more things the team felt they should have done differently.
3. Did the team know where the difficult airway cart/equipment located?
4. Did the team know what is in the difficult airway cart? Is the cart organized and labeled so that it is easy to find what you are looking for?
5. Is the team comfortable with the equipment in the difficult airway cart?
6. Is there a video laryngoscope available?
7. Have the updated American Society of Anesthesiologists Difficult Airway Algorithms available and familiarize the team.
8. Acknowledge that there are differences in each member's approach to a difficult airway situation and the best approach is one that each member is most comfortable with.
9. Stress the need to keep up one's skill with continuing medical education opportunities such as difficult airway workshop, using simulations, and utilizing new supraglottic devices and video laryngoscope in controlled settings.
10. Identify up to three process improvements the facility will develop after the drill which will better equip them for next time.

Discussion

The American Society of Anesthesiologists published the Practice Guidelines for Management of the Difficult Airway in 1993, updating these in 2003 and then again in February 2013 (see Figure 7.1). This latest updated guideline reflected the more recent evaluation of scientific literature and the development and incorporation of many alternative airway devices into clinical practice in the past 10 years.[1] The purpose of the guideline is to facilitate the management of the difficult airway and to reduce the likelihood of adverse outcome by providing an organized algorithm, starting with the patient's history and physical evaluation of the airway, strategy for preparation, intubation, and extubation of the difficult airway.[2]

Respiratory adverse events have been reported as the second most adverse intraoperative events occurring in ambulatory surgeries, with an incidence of 0.2–0.5% for intubation-related events such as difficult intubation, esophageal intubation, and dental damages.[3] A recent American Society of Anesthesiologists (ASA) closed claims study, looking at the risks and safety of anesthesia in remote locations from claims from 1990 or later, showed that when compared to the operation room claims, 50% of remote location claims occurred with monitored anesthetic care.[4] Gastrointestinal suite was the most common remote location followed by cardiology locations. Remote location claims have a higher severity of injuries. Respiratory damaging events were the most common mechanism of injury in both the operating room and remote location, but when compared with the operating room claims the remote claims for respiratory adverse events were more than double.[4]

The Royal College of Anesthetists and the Difficult Airway Society of the United Kingdom published the fourth National Audit Project (NAP4) in 2011. The project was done to look at and study the major complications of airway management during anesthesia in the UK over a 12-month period. Based on the data collected, the incidence of serious airway complications during general anesthesia is at least one in 22,000 anesthetics.[5] When good or appropriate care is delivered, the risk of death or brain damage is about 1 per million of general anesthetics and the risk of serious injury is 1 in 100,000. Most patients who were injured had received suboptimal care.[6]

Lessons learned from the NAP4:[5,6]

1. Anesthesia providers should perform airway assessment; have a plan and strategy for unanticipated airway difficulty which can be rapidly carried out
2. Not all patients are candidates for using a supraglottic airway (SGA)
3. If an awake fiberoptic intubation (AFOI) is deemed necessary, then it should be used
4. Aspiration is the most common cause of anesthesia airway-related mortality
5. Obese patients are at increased risk of an adverse airway event
6. Cricothyroidotomy by anesthetists is associated with high rate of failure
7. One in four events occurred at the end of anesthesia or in early recovery room
8. Omission or incorrect interpretation of capnography led to esophageal intubation.

Many anesthesia societies worldwide have recommendations and guidelines for the management of the difficult airway.[1,7–9] The common threads among these recommendations and guidelines are as follows:

Preparation

1. Every facility should have readily available at least one portable storage unit that contains specialized equipment for difficult airway management, and the anesthesia providers should be familiar and comfortable with using them
2. Anesthesia providers should be cognizant of the importance of knowledge, technical and nontechnical skills in the management of the airway and keeping these skills up to date
3. Anesthesia providers and the OR team should participate in airway drills and simulation training and incorporate briefing and debriefing of events to the team. Each team member is encouraged to be an active participant and speak up during an adverse airway event
4. A thorough preoperative airway history and exam should be done on every patient prior to the initiation of anesthetic care to predict difficult airway management
5. An airway plan should be discussed with the patient and additional help should be available if needed
6. Supplemental oxygenation is first priority.

Anticipated difficult airway

An anticipated difficult airway is the one in which a conventionally trained anesthesiologist anticipates difficulty with mask ventilation or tracheal intubation or both after a comprehensive history and airway exam. The patient may exhibit certain features on airway exam that may prompt the anesthesiologist to consider that airway management may be difficult. The following steps are recommended for an effective management in case a difficult airway is anticipated.[1]

A patient with an anticipated difficult airway may be managed at an ambulatory surgical center depending on multiple factors such as the nature of needed procedure, system issues of availability of additional skilled help in times of need, and the knowledge and skill level of the providers.

1. Explain in detail to the patient the risks and the methods that will be implemented in airway management
2. Inform the surgeon about concerns of potential difficult airway
3. There should be additional skilled help available in the ambulatory center, as well as arrangement to admit certain patients to a hospital if needed
4. If patient is cooperative, active pre-oxygenation should be provided prior to any intervention and

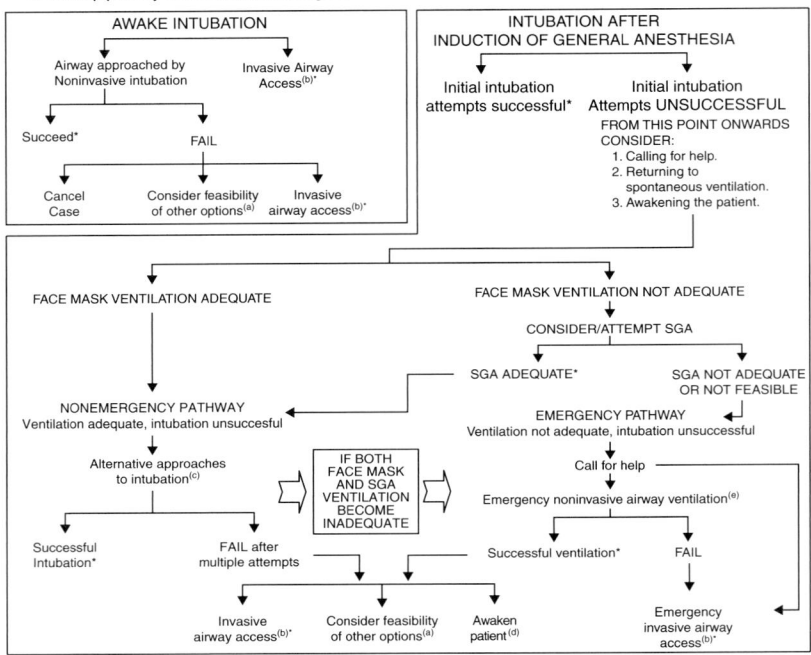

DIFFICULT AIRWAY ALGORITHM

1. Assess the likelihood and clinical impact of basic management problems:
   - Difficulty with patient cooperation or consent
   - Difficult mask ventilation
   - Difficult supraglottic airway placement
   - Difficult laryngoscopy
   - Difficult intubation
   - Difficult surgical airway access

2. Actively pursue opportunities to deliver supplemental oxygen throughout the process of difficult airway management.

3. Consider the relative merits and feasibility of basic management choices:

   - Awake intubation *vs.* intubation after induction of general anesthesia
   - Non-invasive technique *vs.* invasive techniques for the initial approach to intubation
   - Video-assisted laryngoscopy as an initial approach to intubation
   - Preservation *vs.* ablation of spontaneous ventilation

4. Develop primary and alternative strategies:

*Confirm ventilation, tracheal intubation, or SGA placement with exhaled CO_2.

Figure 7.1 Difficult Airway Algorithm from the American Society of Anesthesiologists. Reprinted with permission[1]

also during management of airway by either a nasal cannula, face mask, or insufflation

5. Every provider should know where the portable airway cart with back-up equipment is located and how to use it

6. The provider should make a decision whether an intubation should be performed awake using a fiberoptic bronchoscope or general anesthesia should be induced prior to intubation. An awake intubation is preferred in predicted cases of difficult predicted supraglottic device placement or difficult mask ventilation

7. Maintenance of spontaneous respirations is helpful if difficult mask ventilation is also predicted

8. A video laryngoscope should be used as an initial approach to intubation, which may provide better outcomes than a conventional direct laryngoscopy; an intubating stylet or gum elastic bougie may be used as an aid to intubation

9. A detailed documentation provided to the patient and on the patient's chart regarding the methods that were successful in management of airway, to aid with subsequent anesthesia encounters.

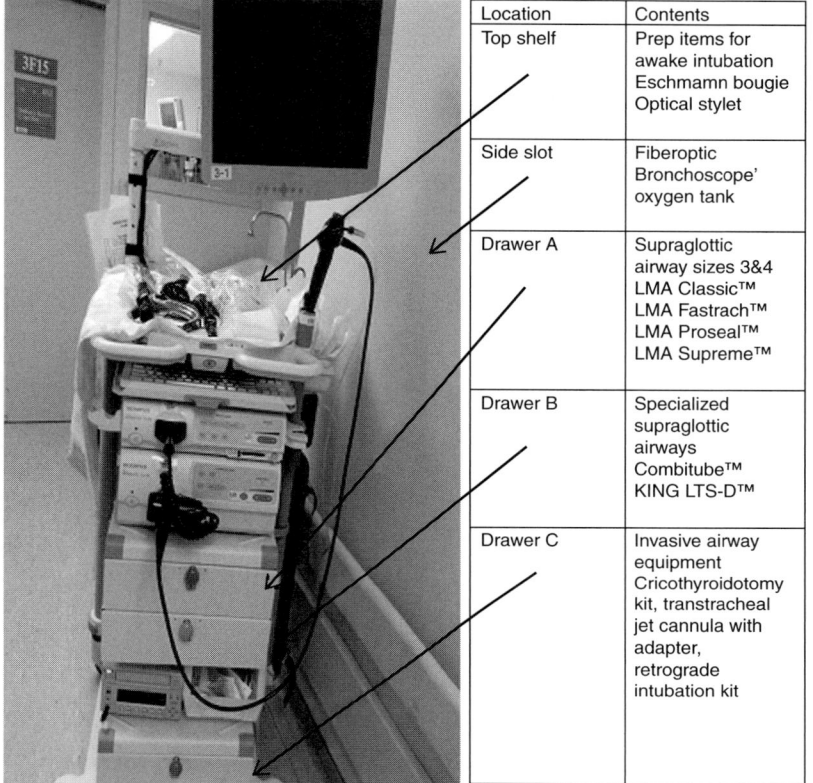

Location	Contents
Top shelf	Prep items for awake intubation Eschmamn bougie Optical stylet
Side slot	Fiberoptic Bronchoscope' oxygen tank
Drawer A	Supraglottic airway sizes 3&4 LMA Classic™ LMA Fastrach™ LMA Proseal™ LMA Supreme™
Drawer B	Specialized supraglottic airways Combitube™ KING LTS-D™
Drawer C	Invasive airway equipment Cricothyroidotomy kit, transtracheal jet cannula with adapter, retrograde intubation kit

Figure 7.2 Example of difficult airway cart: Color-coded drawers

Unanticipated difficult airway

An unanticipated difficult airway adds an element of surprise after induction of anesthesia in a situation where either mask ventilation is inadequate or an intubation may be difficult in the presence of adequate mask ventilation ("cannot intubate, cannot ventilate scenario").[1,10]

Recommended steps for management of this unanticipated situation are as follows:

1. Actively pursue means to provide supplemental oxygenation, which can be achieved via nasal cannula or a facemask
2. If difficulty is encountered after induction with mask ventilation, place either an oral or nasopharyngeal airway to rule out airway obstruction as a potential cause for difficult ventilation
3. Call for help and difficult airway cart, attempt two-handed mask ventilation
4. Place a supraglottic device such as an LMA to provide ventilation and a possible conduit for intubation
5. Call for a fiberoptic bronchoscope or video laryngoscope
6. Consider waking up the patient if able to adequately ventilate and oxygenate
7. If a situation is "cannot ventilate, cannot intubate", prepare for a possible surgical airway such as cricothyroidotomy or tracheostomy
8. A rigid bronchoscope should be available
9. Patient should be extubated when fully awake
10. A detailed documentation provided to the patient and on their chart regarding the methods that were successful in airway management, to aid with subsequent anesthesia encounters.

Extubation of difficult airway

The NAP4 study showed that 30% of adverse airway events occurred during emergence and in or during transfer to the recovery room.[5] The ASA closed claims data revealed that 12% of difficult airway events occurred on extubation and 5% during recovery.[11] Given the high risk of adverse airway events during

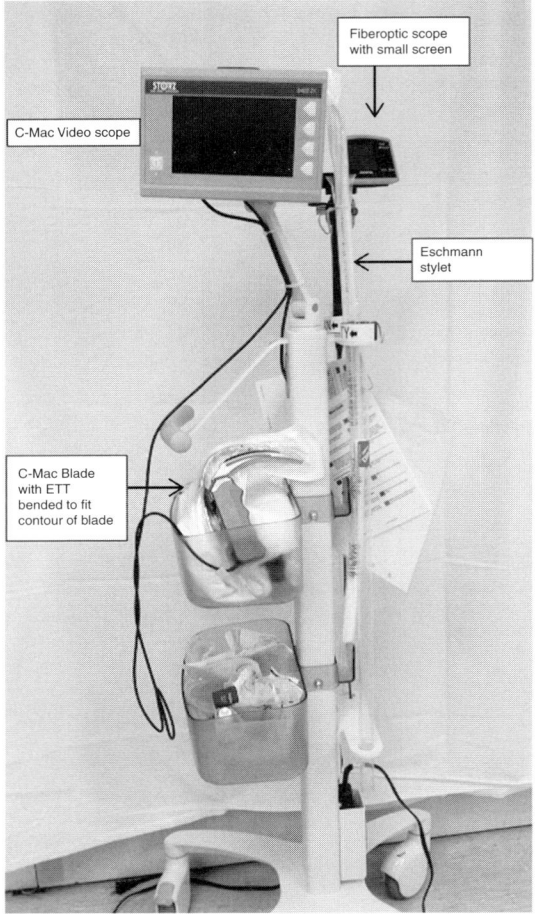

Figure 7.3 Example of portable difficult airway cart

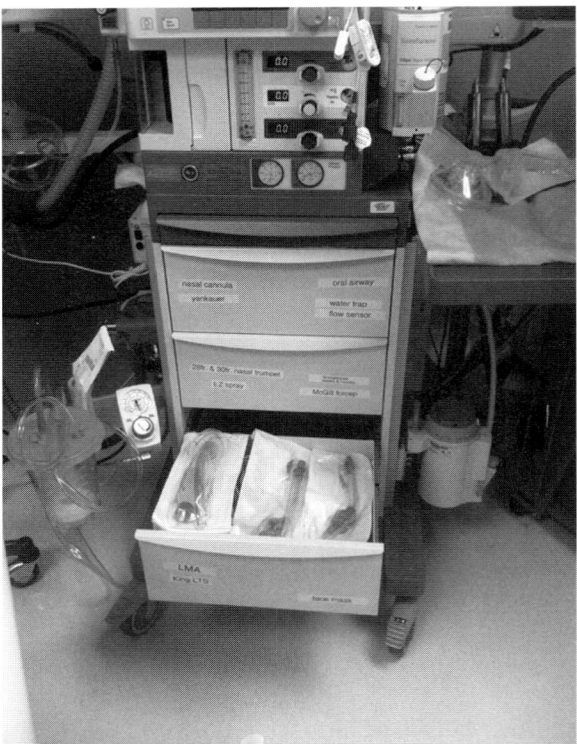

Figure 7.4 Example of anesthesia machine with LMAs and laryngeal tubes in drawer

emergence and extubation, the anesthesia provider should have an extubation plan.

1. Evaluate the risk of difficult intubation, reintubation, access to the airway, and available resources if patient cannot maintain oxygenation and ventilation when extubated
2. Consider the need to remain intubated postoperatively and transport to a hospital for ICU admission
3. Plan for an awake extubation
4. Strategies for extubation using an airway exchange catheter:
   – This hollow stylet is inserted into the endotracheal tube (ETT) to a predetermined length so that it is in the trachea but does not pass the carina
   – Certain airway exchange catheters can be connected to the anesthesia circuit or self-inflating ventilation bag, so passive oxygenation can be given if needed
   – If patient is awake and maintaining oxygenation and ventilation, the catheter can be removed
   – If reintubation is required, an ETT can be placed over the airway exchange catheter and guided down to the trachea blindly or with the assistance of direct laryngoscopy, fiberoptic, or videoscopy
5. Extubation using laryngeal mask airway (LMAs such as Classic, Unique, or Intubating) or air-Q supraglottic device:
   – LMAs may be used as a bridge for extubation
   – LMAs acting as supraglottic ventilation to reduce hemodynamic stress, coughing, or bucking
   – LMAs can be used as a conduit for reintubation using a fiberoptic scope.

Follow-up of a difficult airway encounter[12]

1. A detailed documentation delineating the steps taken to ventilate, oxygenate, and intubate should be noted on the patient's chart

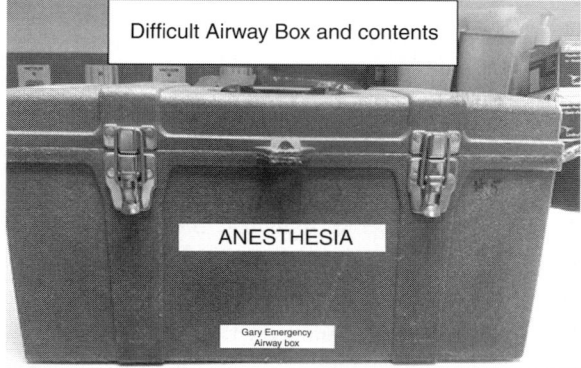

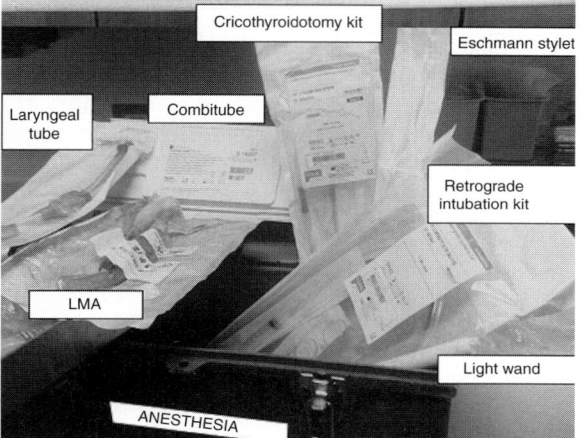

Figure 7.5 Example of difficult airway box and contents

2. A difficult airway alert should be acknowledged on the electronic medical record if available
3. Patient should be given a letter with detailed information about the difficult airway encounter
4. Patient should be advised to obtain a medical bracelet and register with a medical alert database such as MedicAlert.

Sample of a difficult airway letter and technical description

Date
 Dear Sir:
 This letter and the accompanying technical description contain important information about you that was discovered during your recent surgery. Please keep it in a safe place. If you drive a car, I suggest that you make a copy of both documents and place them in the glove compartment of your car.

Before you undergo any type of operation in which anesthesia or sedation is used, your surgeon and anesthesiologist should read this letter. You should also show it to your primary care physician. He or she will be able to advise you if other health care providers should have access to this information before they administer special treatments to you. Please register with a medical alert database indicating that you have a difficult airway and obtain a medical alert bracelet to be worn at all times.

The reason for writing this letter is as follows: In the process of giving you anesthesia for your recent operation, we found it difficult to insert an endotracheal tube (breathing tube) into your trachea (the windpipe that carries air to your lungs). This is a relatively rare condition and one that is often difficult to predict. Knowing about this condition in advance will help your physicians plan the safest possible treatments, and will minimize the chance of associated hazards and complications.

If you or your health care providers have any questions about this letter, please do not hesitate to call at any time. The office phone number is (   ). The remainder of this letter is a technical description of your problem that may be helpful to anesthesiologists and other health care providers.
 Sincerely,
 Name of the institution
 Anesthesiology Department

DIFFICULT INTUBATION DESCRIPTION

Patient Name: _____ Date of Surgery _____
Surgical
Procedure_____
Anesthesiologist_____
Name of the hospital or surgical center_____

PHYSICAL DATA:

Habitus: Height: Weight:
Mouth opening (cm):
Mallampatti class: I   II   III   IV
Thyromental distance   < 6 cm   >6 cm
Hyomental distance
Range of neck motion: limited/full
Neck circumference:
Facial anomalies:_____
Teeth:_____

MASK AIRWAY:

Qualitative description (circle)   easy   difficult
Airway support devices (circle)
   oral airway   nasal airway   head strap
Other mask airway comments:
   one-handed   two-handed
Supraglottic devices:_____

LARYNGOSCOPY:

Laryngoscopy technique with a rigid blade
(specify type and size) _____
Associated with successful fiberoptic scope
Videoscope (specify)
Extent of cord visualization: (Cormack–Lehane
Grade)   I   II   III   IV
Other laryngoscopy: comments:

INTUBATION:

Was intubation successful   Yes   No
Successful intubation while: awake   asleep
Blind intubation   Yes   No
Successful intubation route: Oral   Nasal
Other intubation
comments:_____

Examples of available difficult airway equipment are shown in Figures 7.2–7.5.

References

1. Apfelbaum JL, Hagberg CA, Caplan RA, et al. Practice guidelines for management of the difficult airway: an updated report by the American Society of Anesthesiologists Task Force on the management of the difficult airway. *Anesthesiology* 2013;118(2):251–270.
2. Hagberg C. ASA difficult airway management guidelines: what's new? *ASA Newsletter* 2013;77(9):10–12.
3. Chung F, Mezei G. Adverse outcomes in ambulatory anesthesia. *Can J Anaesth* 1999;46(5):R18–R26.
4. Metzner J, Posner K, Domino K. The risk and safety of anesthesia at remote locations: the US closed claims analysis. *Curr Opin Anaesthesiol* 2009;22(4):502–508.
5. Cook T, Woodall N, Frerk C. Major complications of airway management in the UK: results of the Fourth National Audit Project of the Royal College of Anaesthetists and the Difficult Airway Society. Part 1: Anaesthesia. *Br J Anaesth* 2011;106:617–631.
6. Anderson J, Klock Jr A. Airway Management. *Anesth Clin N Am* 2014;32:445–461.
7. Law J, Broemling N, Cooper R, Drolet P, Duggan L, et al. The difficult airway with recommendation for management- Part 1- Difficult tracheal intubation encountered in an unconscious/induced patient. *Can J Anaesth* 2013;60:1089–1118.
8. Law J, Broemling N, Cooper R, Drolet P, Duggan L, et al. The difficult airway with recommendations for management- Part 2- The anticipated difficult airway. *Can J Anaesth* 2013;60:1119–1138.
9. Mellanby E, Podmore B, McNary A. Safety in the emergency situation: the airway – a theatre team approach. *J Periop Pract* 2014;24(5):112–117.
10. Greenland K. Difficult airway management in an ambulatory surgical center? *Curr Opin Anaesthesiol* 2012;25:659–664.
11. Metzner J, Posner K, Lam M, Domino K. Closed claims analysis. *Best Pract Res Clin Anaesthesiol* 2011;25:263–276.
12. Popat M, Mitchell V, Dravid R, Patel A, Swampillai C, Higgs A. Difficult Airway Society Guidelines for the management of tracheal extubation. *Anaesthesia* 2012;67(3):318–340.

Chapter

8

Local anesthetic systemic toxicity

Niraja Rajan and Steven Butz

Introduction

Local anesthetics are widely used in surgical facilities by a variety of healthcare providers.

The three scenarios presented here deal with different situations and mechanisms by which local anesthetic systemic toxicity (LAST) may present in a patient.

Careful preparation, attention to detail, and vigilance go a long way in the prevention, early detection, and management of LAST.

Educational objectives

1. Take steps to prevent LAST
2. Recognize early signs and symptoms of LAST
3. Effectively manage LAST.

Scenario 1: LAST in a patient receiving a regional block

A 48-year-old male presents for shoulder arthroscopy and rotator cuff repair.

He has a history of hyperlipidemia and takes atorvastatin. He denies chest pain or dyspnea. He has had previous uncomplicated general anesthetics. He is a non-smoker and has a BMI of 33.

The anesthetic plan was general anesthesia with an interscalene block for postoperative pain management. The block was performed in the preoperative holding area under ultrasound and nerve stimulator guidance, with 30 ml of 1% ropivacaine.

Now the patient complains of "feeling funny", light-headedness, metallic taste, and anxiety. Vital signs: HR has increased from 82 to 110; BP increased from 110/70 to 150/90; SpO_2 has remained 99%.

Expected actions:

1. Call for help if needed
2. Anticipate seizures and take steps to prevent and treat them
3. Monitor for worsening signs of local anesthetic toxicity
4. Airway management/supplemental oxygen.

Scenario continued:

After group has assembled, PVCs are noted on the monitor. It progresses over the next 2 min to widening QRS complexes and he has lost consciousness.

Expected actions:

1. Call for help
2. Check for pulse
3. Anticipate cardiac arrest
4. Airway management and ventilation.

Scenario continued:

There is no pulse.

Expected actions:

1. Begin CPR and ACLS protocol for pulseless ventricular tachycardia/ventricular fibrillation. *CPR needs to be continued throughout administration of medications until pulse is restored*
2. Advanced airway management. Intubation is indicated for patients undergoing CPR. *Alternative methods of oxygenation may be used if personnel with intubation skills are unavailable*
3. Administer vasopressors as needed
4. Call for intralipid

Perioperative Drill-Based Crisis Management, ed. Steven Butz. Published by Cambridge University Press. © Cambridge University Press 2016.

5. In a freestanding facility, 9-1-1 services should be activated. In a hospital with a code team, a code system should be activated to mobilize additional resources
6. Use cognitive aids when available (ACLS algorithm, ASRA guidelines).

Scenario continued:

The drill would end when the participants administer 20% intralipid.

Scenario 2: LAST in OR from drug swap

An 11-year-old, 56 kg patient is in the operating room for an anterior cruciate ligament (ACL) repair. The patient and family elected to have a femoral nerve catheter placed for postoperative pain relief. The patient is an avid soccer player and takes insulin for his type 1 diabetes. He has never previously had anesthesia. Glucose preoperatively is 111 mg/dl. A paternal uncle had an "allergy" to general anesthesia for which he had to go to the ICU postoperatively. The family doesn't know any other details and neither parent has had general anesthesia, but the father was warned to avoid general anesthesia.

The plan is to place the catheter after the induction of general anesthesia by mask. The catheter is placed using a combination of nerve stimulation and ultrasound. There are some technical difficulties, but the catheter is placed after 30 min and many attempts to create the potential space using 30 ml of 0.2% ropivacaine.

The patient is prepped and draped when there is tachycardia to 168 beats per minute noted on the monitor.

Expected actions:

1. Assess patient and verify functioning of equipment
2. Assure ventilation and oxygenation
3. Differential diagnosis of pain, light anesthesia, tachyarrhythmia of cardiac etiology, anaphylaxis, malignant hyperthermia, LAST
4. Perform actions that may eliminate possibilities such as skin exam, analyze a printed ECG strip, listen for wheezing, check end tidal carbon dioxide.

Scenario continued:

The circulating nurse in the room realizes that 30 ml of 0.5% ropivacaine was used instead of 0.2% ropivacaine. The monitor now shows a wide QRS with a rate of 35 bpm.

Expected actions:

1. Call for help and retrieve code cart
2. Check for adequate perfusion and begin CPR if insufficient
3. Begin ACLS for ventricular tachycardia with pulse
4. Prepare and administer 20% lipid emulsion
5. Consider prophylactic seizure treatment with benzodiazepines.

Scenario continued:

Patient after a round of CPR and ACLS now has asystole.

Expected actions:

1. Continue treatment along ACLS protocol for asystole
2. Arrange for transportation to facility with cardiopulmonary bypass availability
3. Give additional lipid emulsion.

Scenario continued:

The drill ends with death or resuscitation that continues in transport to hospital with bypass availability.

Scenario 3: Delayed LAST in recovery room

A 48-year-old man is scheduled for a left ACL reconstruction under general anesthesia and femoral/sciatic nerve block. He has a history of hepatitis C and is being followed by his gastroenterologist. Recent liver function tests are stable, with mildly elevated serum transaminases and normal coagulation studies. The rest of the history and clinical examination is unremarkable. His weight is 70 kg and BMI is 26.

Expected actions:

1. Keep decreased liver function in mind while calculating the dose of local anesthetic for the nerve block
2. Discuss these concerns with the surgical team.

Scenario continued:

The patient undergoes an uneventful femoral/sciatic nerve block in the preoperative area, with 0.5% bupivacaine (total volume 35 ml). The surgery proceeds uneventfully. At the end of the 2 h procedure, the surgeon injects 30 ml of 0.5% bupivacaine into and around the knee joint.

Expected actions:

1. The surgical team should discuss the need for additional local anesthetic with the anesthesia team

2. The surgical and anesthesia team should be in agreement about the allowable maximum limit of local anesthetic drug in the patient.

Scenario continued:

The patient is transported to the recovery room. About 30 min into recovery, the patient complains of feeling anxious and lightheaded.

Expected actions:

1. Inform the anesthesia team
2. Monitor vital signs
3. Assess pain level
4. Supplemental O_2.

Scenario continued:

The anesthesia provider is at the bedside. PVCs are noted on the patient monitor. HR 120 s; SpO_2 98%; non-invasive blood pressure (NIBP) 160/90. Over the next 5 min, QRS widening is observed which progressively deteriorates to ventricular tachycardia.

Expected actions:

1. Check for pulse/responsiveness
2. Call for help
3. Get the code cart.

Scenario continued:

The patient has a pulse, NIBP 156/84, and he is responsive.

Expected actions:

1. Follow the ACLS ventricular tachycardia with a pulse algorithm
2. Consider differential diagnoses
3. Consider the potential for LAST
4. Start intralipid 20%.

Scenario continued:

The rhythm will normalize after the infusion of 20% intralipid.

Expected actions:

1. Discharge/transfer planning
2. Discuss the importance of communication.

Debriefing

1. Identify up to three or more things the team felt went well with the scenario.
2. Identify up to three or more things the team felt they should have done differently.

3. What equipment was difficult to locate or use?
4. Could staff find 20% lipid emulsion or did someone try to use propofol instead?
5. What was missing, that the facility would need, to fully care for the patient?
6. If presented with a similar case what would the staff do differently next time?
7. Convey the lessons learned from *this particular case*, and generalize them so they can apply the lesson to other, real-life situations.
8. Correct facts that you know are incorrect, but acknowledge controversies where there are different styles but the BEST approach is not really known.
9. Good debriefing takes a lot of practice and feedback to master. Work with a partner and give each other feedback specifically about your debriefing skills whenever possible.
10. Stress the importance of asking for and using cognitive aids (algorithms).
11. Identify up to three process improvements the facility will develop after the drill that will better equip them for next time.

Discussion

The American Society of Regional Anesthesia and Pain Medicine provides a practice advisory for local anesthetic systemic toxicity (LAST) published in 2010 and updated in 2012.[2,5] LAST can be the result of an inadvertent direct intravascular injection of local anesthetic or from absorption of local anesthetic from the site of injection when a very large dose has been used.

Systemic toxicity after injection of local anesthetic tends to be more common in females and patients over 60 years of age or under 16. Ninety percent of LAST occurs with the use of bupivacaine, ropivacaine, and levo-bupivacaine. More than a third of patients have an underlying cardiac, metabolic, hepatic, or renal disease.

The timing of onset of symptoms in cases of direct intravascular injection averages 52 s from the time of injection. Most case reports give an onset of symptoms at 1–5 min post injection, but 25% had onset greater than 5 min with one report describing a 60 min delay. Delayed onset of symptoms probably represents systemic absorption from the injection site as opposed to direct intravascular injection.

The classic symptoms involve the CNS and range from excitatory symptoms to seizures to CNS depression. Initial symptoms may be metallic taste or auditory symptoms, but also psychiatric changes or agitation. The cardiac symptoms typically occur shortly after the

61

CNS symptoms and follow the same pattern of excitation to depression. Initially hypertension and tachycardia may be seen with arrhythmias. This is followed by cardiac depression and cardiovascular collapse. Bupivacaine results in cardiac toxicity at plasma levels that produce CNS toxicity, unlike other local anesthetics which produce CNS toxicity first, and then cardiac toxicity at much higher plasma levels. This means that if a patient experiences CNS symptoms following bupivacaine injection, circulatory collapse is not far behind.

Necessary steps to minimize the likelihood of intravascular injection that are supported in the literature include:

1. Use the lowest possible drug volume and concentration to achieve effect. This reduces the total amount of drug given (dose x concentration)
2. Do not exceed maximum allowed dose of local anesthetic. These levels have been calculated for different local anesthetic agents based on plasma levels at which CNS toxicity would result if the drug was injected IV. It is important to calculate the maximum safe dose of local anesthetic for a patient before proceeding with regional anesthesia or local infiltration by the surgeon. Remember that different local anesthetic agents have additive toxicities. Therefore local anesthetic agents administered in the surgical field, in addition to the regional anesthetic, could result in additive toxicity. Keep patient comorbidities and age in mind when calculating maximum allowed doses for local anesthetics
3. Use incremental doses (of 3–5 ml) with pauses in between doses. Pauses should reflect the circulation time, but keeping the needle fixed may be difficult and more rapid administration may be indicated. The balance between waiting and needle movement may be less important with ultrasound guidance as the needle can often be moved purposefully with this technique
4. Aspirate prior to injection; however, there is a 2% false-negative rate with this technique
5. When injecting potentially toxic doses of local anesthetic, use of an intravascular marker such as epinephrine is recommended.

Use of ultrasound guidance has not been shown to reduce the likelihood of LAST in human studies or reports.[4]

Treatment of LAST should be as follows:

1. Airway management should be primary during the initial manifestation of LAST, as hypoxia and acidosis potentiate LAST

2. If seizure occurs, treatment begins with benzodiazepines. Propofol or thiopental may also be used, but these have greater cardiac depressant effects
3. If seizures persist, consider neuromuscular blockade to minimize acidosis created by muscular lactic acid formation. This does not stop seizures and sedation *must* still be administered
4. ACLS protocols are modified for LAST:
   a. Reduce dose of epinephrine
   b. *Do not* give calcium channel blockers or beta-blockers
   c. *Do not* treat arrhythmias with local anesthetics
   d. Amiodarone is the anti-arrhythmic of choice
5. Lipid emulsion 20% should be used at the initial signs of LAST, following airway management.[1] Propofol *does not* replace lipid emulsion as it has lower lipid content and can potentiate myocardial depression.
   a. 1.5 ml/kg 20% lipid emulsion bolus
   b. 0.25 ml/kg/min of infusion, continued for at least 10 min after circulatory stability is attained
   c. If circulatory stability is not attained, consider a repeat bolus and increasing infusion to 0.5 ml/kg/min
   d. Approximately 10 ml/kg lipid emulsion for 30 min is recommended as the upper limit for initial dosing
6. If no response to treatment, placement on cardiopulmonary bypass is the last option
7. ASRA has issued an updated version of the checklist for the management of LAST.[3,5] Electronic copies of the ASRA checklist, for lamination and inclusion in a local anesthetic toxicity kit, are available from the ASRA website (www.asra.com).

References

1. Neal et al. ASRA practice advisory on local anesthetic systemic toxicity. *Reg Anesth Pain Med* (2010) 35(2): 152–161.
2. Neal JM, Mulroy MF, Weinberg GL; American Society of Regional Anesthesia and Pain Medicine checklist for managing local anesthetic systemic toxicity: 2012 version. *Reg Anesth Pain Med* (2012) 37(1):16–18.
3. Salinas FV, Hanson NA. Evidence-based medicine for ultrasound-guided regional anesthesia. *Anesthesiol Clin* (2014) 32(4):771–787.
4. www.lipidrescue.org
5. Neal et al. ASRA checklist improves trainee performance during a simulated episode of local anesthetic systemic toxicity. *Reg Anesth Pain Med* (2012) 37(1): 8–15.

Violence in the workplace
An active shooter in an ASC

Deborah S. Lowery

Introduction

Most healthcare facilities have emergency action plans (EAPs) for medical emergencies, natural and environmental disasters, and fire safety. An EAP for violence in the workplace, specifically an active shooter event, is increasingly becoming a topic for consideration for all types of healthcare facilities.

An active shooter, by definition agreed upon by multiple U.S. government agencies, is "*an individual actively engaged in killing or attempting to kill people in a confined space and populated area*."[1]

According to research from Johns Hopkins, performed in the aftermath of an active shooter event at their medical center, shootings in the healthcare setting are still relatively rare in the overall context of workplace violence.[2] However, a recent report published by the FBI and Texas State University also indicates an increasing annual frequency of active shooter incidents, and thereby causalities[1] (see Figures 9.1 and 9.2).

This report elucidates that mass casualties can occur in a matter of minutes, with most incidents lasting five minutes or less. The FBI has concluded that "even when law enforcement was present or able to respond within minutes, civilians often had to make life and death decisions, and therefore, should be engaged in training and discussions on decisions they may face."[1] This would indicate the need for and promotion of a measured, proactive response to devising an active shooter response plan for your ASC.

Although not as easily translatable to uniform pre-established drill formats as medical events, active shooter response preparation and practice can encompass many options. These can include: education, PowerPoint, and roundtable discussions; watching videos of staged presentations by various institutions that already have established active shooter response plans in place; and/or conducting drills that are site-specific and tailored to one's unique physical layout and resources.

The Department of Homeland Security and FEMA websites provide online educational courses that could be part of continuing education.[3,5,6]

The scenarios presented here, though generic, encompass many of the concepts that need to be understood, remembered, and considered when confronted with an active shooter situation. Recommendations for appropriate ("best") responses are taken from current thinking of experts in the field, both from the government and private sectors.

Educational objectives

1. Identify and understand common characteristics of an active shooter in an effort to quickly assess situation and level of danger
2. Become familiar with the most recent knowledge, profiles and trends of active shooter incidents to aid in making critical decisions
3. Adopt and execute the survival mindset training to quickly determine the most reasonable way(s) to protect your own life
4. Gain understanding of the components involved in selecting a strategy for response:
   – Evacuate
   – Alert others
   – Inform law enforcement
   – Hide out with lockdown and barricade if cannot evacuate
   – Take counteraction as last resort
5. Understand that these phases can act together or separately. Implementation does not require you

Perioperative Drill-Based Crisis Management, ed. Steven Butz. Published by Cambridge University Press. © Cambridge University Press 2016.

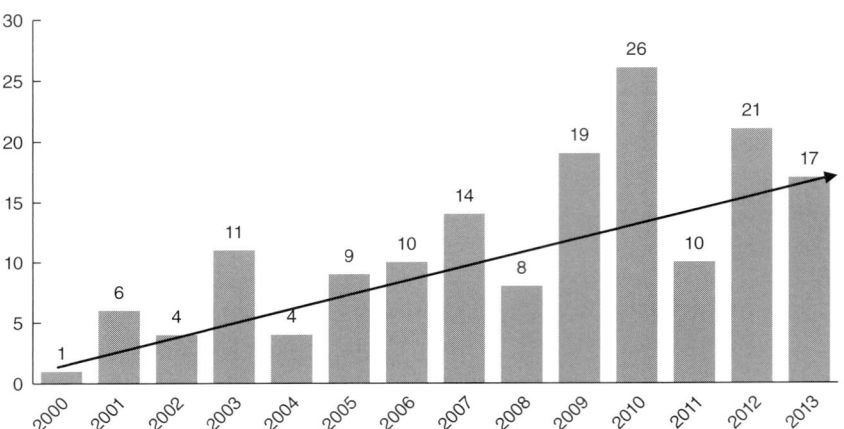

Figure 9.1 A study of 160 active shooter incidents in the United States, 2000–2013: Incidents annually[1]

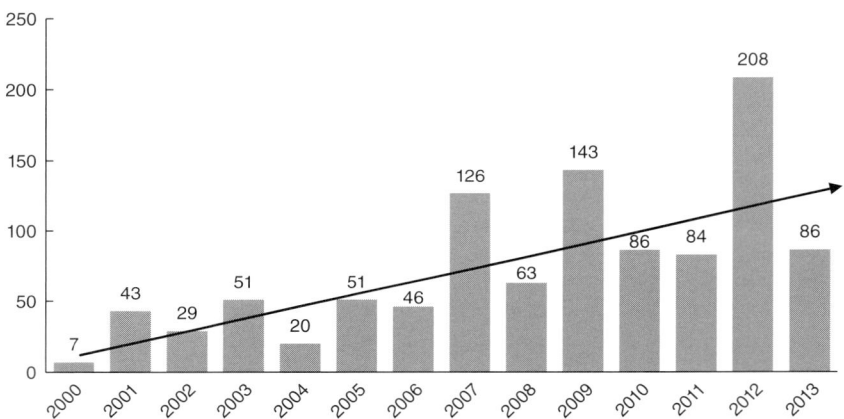

Figure 9.2 A study of 160 active shooter incidents in the United States, 2000–2013: Annual totals of 1043 casualties[1]

to work sequentially or include all of these phases, although *always* alert and inform

6. Know what to do when law enforcement arrives
7. Employ prevention: Recognize warning signs or indicators of potential violence by an employee or co-worker and institute remediation or mitigation.

Scenario 1: Active shooter in a freestanding setting

Takes place in a freestanding multi-level ASC building with the registration and surgical area on the ground floor, located immediately inside the entry way to either side of the lobby.

A nurse is escorting a patient and her husband from registration into the busy preop holding area where several patients are already in bays in various stages of preparation: undressing, being interviewed, or getting IVs placed. As the entry door closes, there is screaming and what sounds like gunshots being fired on the other side of that door. The door is one that needs to be "badged in" so, for the immediate time, it is secured.

Expected actions:

1. Recognize the sounds as gunshots. Not infrequently these sounds are misinterpreted or rationalized as "fireworks", "cars backfiring", or "construction noises"
2. Assume the worst; understand the severity and the need to make quick decisions
3. Expect confused responses and anticipate chaos

4. Decide that *evacuation* is an acceptable option in this situation
5. Know options for escape route(s) and direct and help others, if possible
6. *Alert* as many as possible in vicinity, loudly and clearly in simple, plain language, to potential life-threatening situation.

Scenario continued:

Nurses from each bay emerge to the shouting and quickly try to shepherd patients and family members towards the exit farthest away from danger. That exit leads to the parking lot. Many are confused and trying to grab clothes, bags; some are refusing to move and are "frozen", some are uncomprehending; one young nurse is hysterical, trying to crawl underneath a cart.

Expected actions:

1. Leave all belongings (your's and patients') behind. Leave with gowns, disconnect monitors, pull out or take IVs, use carts, wheelchairs, do whatever is necessary to move people the fastest
2. Use any additional means to *inform* if the situation allows: PA system, panic button, intercom, hospital operator or security
3. Be authoritative and persuasive with others, compel to evacuate, help as situation allows, but evacuate regardless if others agree to follow
4. Call 911 as soon as safely possible. Be calm, clear, and concise. Give as much information as you can.

Scenario continued:

At this point, the nurse manager is calling 911 but the only information she is able to report is location of the active shooter, locations of other potential victims in the building, and where her group is exiting. Also, as people are leaving the building, a group of residents is coming towards the door. Sirens are heard as police cars are pulling up into the parking lot where people are running out.

Expected actions:

1. Warn and prevent anyone else from entering the area or building
2. Understand that law enforcement arriving can be from multiple sources, therefore dressed differently and with various weapons and even body armor
3. Remain calm and follow officers' instructions

4. Put down anything you might still have in your hands
5. Immediately raise hands and spread fingers and instruct others to do the same. *Keep hands visble at all times*
6. Avoid pointing, screaming, yelling, or making quick movements
7. As the situation allows, try to account for individuals, determining whether anyone is missing or needs additional help
8. Assess psychological state of individuals and provide comfort.

Scenario continued:

Drill ends as law enforcement enters building and evacuated group moves to safer zone. It turns out that the shooter was the estranged husband of a registration clerk, a victim of domestic abuse who had recently filed for divorce and child custody. Victims included the lobby receptionist, the clerk, and two patients who were registering for surgery. The shooter then turned the gun on himself as law enforcement arrived through the front entrance.

Scenario 2: Active shooter in a freestanding center

On a busy afternoon in a freestanding ASC, six operating rooms (ORs) are currently in use. The charge nurse is in the OR corridor and hears yelling coming from the Director of Nursing's office, which is located just steps away. She recognizes the angry voice of a surgical nurse who was fired last week; he had called many of his colleagues over the weekend to elicit support, but without success. As the charge nurse walks toward the office to help, she hears deafening gunshots at close range. Unsure of her ability to exit before the gunman comes out of office, the charge nurse takes cover in the nearest OR, where surgery is taking place.

Expected actions:

1. *Alert* and *inform* as many people as possible, including the other ORs, in plain, simple language that an active shooter is nearby, where and with whom
2. *Call 911* as soon as feasible: give clear, concise information about: location, and if known, identity of shooter(s), physical description, number and/or type of weapons, number of potential victims, and

where they are located. If you cannot speak, leave the line open, if possible, to allow the dispatcher to listen

3. All personnel quickly recognize the threat and move to *lock down* the areas as it is perceived too risky to evacuate safely

4. Try to get out of shooter's view: close, cover, and stay away from any windows.

5. If possible lock doors and *barricade* with furniture, carts, mobile cabinets, towers, operating microscopes, or any heavy equipment. Consider moving patient to the floor and using the heavy locked OR table to barricade

6. Find *cover* (preferable) or *concealment*

7. Move patient to safest area of room continuing necessary care

8. Use time to prepare other strategies (*counter* or *evacuate*) should the shooter gain entry

9. Identify what could be used as weapons and make a plan to deploy. This could include surgical instruments, chemicals, fire extinguishers, etc.

10. *Silence cell phones and pagers.* Even vibrate settings can give away a hiding position

11. Turn off any sources of noise, including monitors as you are able

12. *Remain quiet!*

Scenario continued:

The shooter is heard moving throughout hallway trying to access the ORs. He is pushing against the door, trying to gain access, firing shots.

Expected actions:

In a last-resort situation where life is in imminent danger:

1. Create noise, movement, *distance* and *distraction* with the intent of decreasing the shooter's accuracy

2. If you cannot flee, try to *incapacitate*

3. *Act as aggressively* as possible

4. Throw items and improvise weapons

5. Yell or scream loudly

6. *Commit to your actions*

Scenario continued:

The drill ends as law enforcement arrives in the OR hallway and exchanges gunfire with the shooter, wounding him and taking him into custody.

Physician and nursing leaders will have to triage and make decisions on how to bring active patient care to a resolution with appropriate transfer to secure the facility. All personnel should be accounted for and assessed for the need for medical or psychological care as law enforcement continues to manage an active crime scene.

Debriefing

1. Identify up to three or more things that were successful in promoting evacuation in the face of a nearby active shooter.

2. Was there an immediate consensus in choice(s) of exits? In retrospect, were they the best choices?

3. What, if any, difficulties were encountered and how could they have been managed better?

4. Identify up to three or more things that were successful in achieving a lockdown–barricade response.

5. Was there the ability to alert and inform others as well as call 911? What available methods were used? Could this have been done differently or better?

6. Were participants able to assume a survival mentality?

7. When in lockdown, were participants able to barricade the room and conceal themselves as effectively as possible? Could anything have been done differently?

8. When in lockdown, could participants work as a team to identify potential weapons for taking action and aggressively countering an active shooter as a last resort? What were they?

9. When encountering law enforcement's arrival, did all participants respond by dropping any items, raising hands, and spreading fingers while remaining calm?

Discussion

After experiencing a hospital shooting at their institution, Johns Hopkins University and School of Medicine published a comprehensive review study that sought to determine and characterize hospital shootings. In *Hospital-Based Shootings in the United States: 2000–2011*, the authors identified and analyzed 154 hospital-related shootings in 40 states. They concluded that, although shootings were "relatively rare compared with other forms of workplace violence", shooters were determined and victims were highly targeted. The overall fatality rate was 57% excluding perpetrator suicides.[2]

A recent joint effort between the FBI and Texas State University resulted in the September 2014 government publication of a report entitled *A Study of Active Shooter Incidents in the United States Between 2000 and 2013* [1] This study specifically referenced healthcare facilities as one of its distinct location categories in the 160 active shooter incidents analyzed. The appendix of this report provides details for the four incidents that took place in that category. Although healthcare settings represent the lowest occurrence rate (2.5%) of active shooter events, the increasing annual frequency of these incidents and the rapid evolution of catastrophic results, many of which occur prior to law enforcement's arrival, reinforce the need for aggressive civilian education and training to hopefully effect a better response and increase the chance for survival.

Characteristics of an active shooter[1,3,4]

- Active shooter: *"An individual(s) actively engaged in killing or attempting to kill people in a confined and populated area"*[1]
- Mostly male (only 3.8% female)
- Mostly single shooter
- Not always a pattern or method to victim selection
- Use of firearm(s); multiple weapons, large amounts of ammo, possible intelligent electronic devices
- Typically mentally ill; holds grudges; acts out against real or perceived injustices; ideologist
- Often on a "pathway to violence" including action plans and access to weapons; and committed to exacting revenge on person(s) or organization
- A new paradigm since September 11, 2001 ("9/11"): offenders often have no real "escape plan." Suicide is common (40%), often welcome "suicide by cop"
- Does not typically involve a "police negotiation" as in a hostage situation as hostage taking is not the purpose of the assault.

Characteristics of ongoing shooting incidents over last 13 years[1]

- Average of 11.4 incidents/year with *increasing trend* (average 16.4/year last 7 years)
- 160 incidents identified by FBI study resulted in 1043 casualties (486 killed/557 wounded)
- 40% fulfill definition of "mass killing": three people or more killed (shooters not included)

- Occurred in 40 states
- All but two were single shooter
- Event is unpredictable, chaotic, evolves quickly: assume great harm can occur before law enforcement's arrival to scene (28% incidents ended <5 min)
- 60% of incidents ended before police arrived
- 13% of incidents were ended by unarmed citizens safely, successfully restraining shooter
- 40% of shooters committed suicide
- 70% occurred in commercial or educational settings
- 2.5% occurred in healthcare facilities.

Many health systems have already put into place education and training programs, as well as drills, on active shooter responses. Resources and recommendations have been derived from experts at the U.S. Department of Homeland Security (DHS), the Department of Justice (DOJ), the International Association of Healthcare Security and Safety (IAHSS), the Federal Emergency Management Agency (FEMA), and the Federal Bureau of Investigation (FBI).[5,6,7]

A draft document is being developed by the Healthcare and Public Sector Coordinating Council (HPH SCC): *Active Shooter Planning and Response in a Healthcare Setting* is a comprehensive source that seeks to provide guidance for the unique challenges and ethical considerations specific to the healthcare setting that impact active shooter response planning. Currently under review by a federal inter-agency group, this draft is posted on the homeland security information network (HSIN) for the intent of providing useful information to the public while awaiting publication.[8]

Taken together, these reports reflect a set of common principles and goals to reduce loss of life and facilitate law enforcement response. Although sensitive in nature and possibly uncomfortable to discuss, there is value in education, preplanning, and training.

Additional educational resources are found in the private sector and are listed in the references.[9,10,11] These are not meant to be exclusive or endorsed, but are included as representative of current industry thinking. These websites also have links to YouTube videos that provide additional perspectives and illustrations of important concepts. Many professionals, including those from the IAHSS, promote the consultation of certified healthcare security experts to provide risk assessments and develop site-specific security and response programs.[7]

Like evidence-based medicine, opinions and recommendations regarding institutional and personal responses to an active shooter are dynamic. There is continual review and refinement as increased knowledge of this complex, multifaceted societal problem is obtained. The following responses reflect consensus of those recent publications and resources.

Knowing your options

In an active shooter situation, all involved persons should quickly determine the most reasonable way to protect their own lives, adopting a survival mindset. If you are in harm's way, you will need to decide rapidly the safest course of action based on the scenario that is unfolding. Patients and visitors will likely follow the lead of employees and managers.

Alert and inform

- Use *plain*, *simple*, and *specific* language to inform as many people as possible of the danger (911, public address system, text messaging, email, intercom)
- Call "911": give location, number of shooters, physical descriptions, numbers/types of weapons, and number of potential victims
- Empower as many people as possible to allow them to make decisions about their best options
- Communicate the location of the intruder(s) location and direction of travel in real time
- Site-specific plans should have clear and direct methods to communicate
- Since shooters usually act alone (98%), effective communication could keep shooter off balance and allow for others to evacuate/lockdown/prepare for counter
- Knowledge and commitment to action is the key to survival
- If in lockdown and can't talk with a "911" operator, leave line open

Evacuate. If there is a safe, accessible escape path, attempt to evacuate the premises. When evacuating:

- Have an escape route and plan in mind
- Leave your belongings behind
- Help others escape, if possible, without increasing the danger to yourself

- Evacuate regardless of whether others agree to follow
- Prevent individuals from entering an area where the active shooter may be present
- Do not attempt to move wounded people if doing so increases the potential of harm to you
- Keep your hands raised and visible if you encounter police
- Follow the instructions of police officers
- Call "911" when it is safe to do so.

Hide out – Lockdown – Barricade. If evacuation is not possible, find a place to hide where the active shooter is less likely to find or gain access to you.

- Need semi-secure area from which you can make survival decisions. Traditional lockdown could create readily identifiable targets
- Call "911" if possible – keep an open line
- Resist urge to panic – go into "survival mode"
- Try to get out of shooter's view
- Stay away from and/or cover windows
- Lock the door/barricade the room with furniture or other heavy items
- Hide behind a large item (for example, a cabinet or desk)
- Consider the difference between cover and concealment. Concealment merely hides from view, cover might protect a person from gunfire. Finding cover is preferable
- Prepare for confrontation should the shooter gain access by utilizing items in the area to incapacitate the shooter
- Use time in lockdown to prepare other strategies (counter or evacuate) should shooter gain entry
- Silence cell phones and pagers (even the vibrate setting can give away a hiding position)
- Turn off any other sources of noise
- Remain quiet.

Take action or Counter. As a last resort, and only if your life or the lives of others are in imminent danger, attempt to disrupt and/or incapacitate the active shooter.[4]

- Create noise, scream, throw objects to distract and place distance between yourself and the shooter to lessen the shooter's accuracy
- Use *any* means available and necessary to survive
- Creating a dynamic environment can provide precious seconds needed in order to evacuate safely

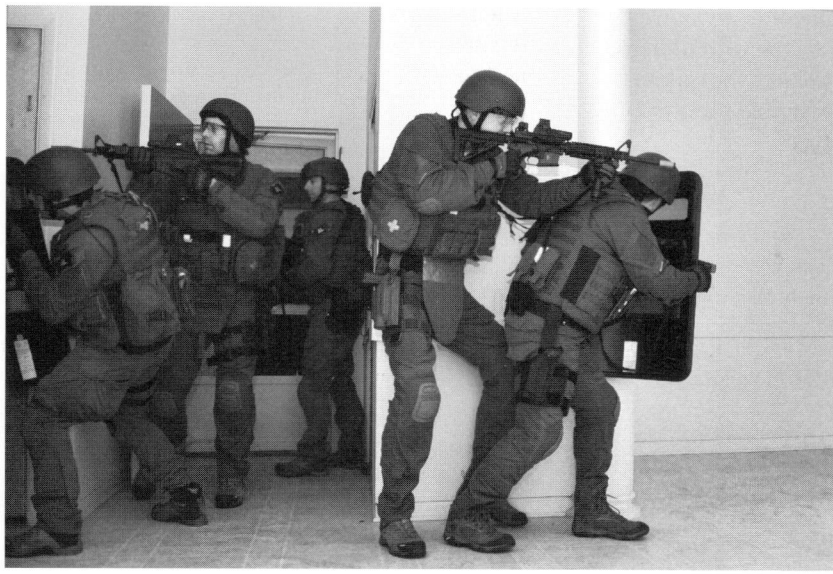

Figure 9.3 Photo courtesy of FBI SWAT US Department of Defense. Photo by John B. Snyder (available under Creative Commons Attribution 4.0 International Public License)

- Work as a team to distract/disarm the shooter if others are present
- Commit to your actions – doing something is better than doing nothing!

When law enforcement arrives[3]

- Remain calm
- Follow officers' instructions
- Immediately raise hands and spread fingers
- Avoid making quick movements towards officers
- Do not grab onto or hold onto officers
- Do not point, yell, or scream
- Do not stop and ask officers for help or directions
- Understand they will not stop to help injured; first priority is to stop event
- Proceed to exit in direction from which the officers are entering.

What about prevention?[3]

- Foster a respectful workplace
- Conduct effective background checks and employee screening.
- Recognize signs or indicators of potential violence by an employee or co-worker that might include:
  - Increased use of alcohol or illegal drugs
  - Increased absenteeism
  - Depression/withdrawal/isolation
  - Mood swings and noticeably unstable emotional responses
  - Increased talk of problems in the home
  - Unsolicited comments about violence, or possessing firearms
- Create a system for reporting signs of potentially violent behavior
- Make counseling available to all employees
- Develop an EAP to include procedures for dealing with an active shooter event
- Implement clear and precise workplace violence policies and procedures
- Conduct workplace violence training regularly.

In conclusion, ambulatory surgery centers, whether freestanding or part of a larger medical establishment, typically have reduced numbers of personnel and limited resources. Often, security or law enforcement is remote or "off-campus" and there are inherent delays in response times for even day-to-day occurrences. An active shooter event is a unique occurrence in which even the most rapid deployment of law enforcement may be insufficient to minimize injuries and fatalities. The additional challenges of caregivers' ethical responsibilities, potential inability to evacuate due to in-progress medical procedures, vulnerable patient populations, presence of hazardous materials, and locked units make this type of disaster planning unique and problematic.[8] Ambulatory surgery centers already have many emergency response plans in place in the event of unanticipated medical and environmental situations. Extending this type of training, vigilance, and preparedness for the unlikely, but potentially catastrophic, experience of an active shooter is prudent.

References

1. Blair, J. Pete, and Schweit, Katherine W. (2014). *A Study of Active Shooter Incidents, 2000–2013*. Texas State University and Federal Bureau of Investigation, U.S. Department of Justice, Washington, DC. http://www.fbi.gov/news/stories/2014/september/fbi-releases-study-on-active-shooter-incidents/pdfs/a-study-of-active-shooter-incidents-in-the-u.s.-between-2000-and-2013 (Accessed May 14, 2015).

2. Kelen, GB, Catlett, CL, et al. (2012) Hospital-based shootings in the United States: 2000–2011. *Annals of Emergency Medicine* 60(6):790–798.

3. U.S. Department of Homeland Security. *Active Shooter How To Respond* www.dhs.gov/xlibrary/assets/active_shooter_booklet.pdf. (Accessed July 11, 2014).

4. U.S. Department of Homeland Security. *Options for Consideration Active Shooter Preparedness Video*. www.dhs.gov/active-shooter-preparedness (Accessed December 6, 2014).

5. U.S. Department of Homeland Security, Office of Infrastructure Protection Webinar. Podcast. Active *Shooter Awarenesss Virtual Roundtable*. www.dhs.gov/active-shooter-preparedness (Accessed December 6, 2014).

6. FEMA Emergency Management Institute (EMI) Independent Study Program Website. *IS-907 Active Shooter: What You Can Do.* (Accessed September 17, 2014).

7. International Association of Healthcare Security and Safety (IAHSS). www.iahss.org (Accessed September 17, 2014).

8. Healthcare and Public Health Sector Coordinating council (HPH SCC). *Active Shooter Planning and Response in a Healthcare Setting.* www.floridahealth.gov (Accessed December 6, 2014).

9. Alice Training Institute. *How to respond to an Active Shooter Event*, www.alicetraining.com (Accessed September 14, 2014).

10. AFIMAC Online Training Academy. www.afimacglobal.com (Accessed October 10, 2014).

11. Mitigation Dynamics Incorporated (MDI). www.mitigationdynamics.com (Accessed October 10, 2014).

Emergency preparedness and evacuation in an ASC

Niraja Rajan and Deborah S. Lowery

Introduction

All ambulatory surgery centers (ASCs), by mandate of the various accreditation agencies as well as Centers for Medicare and Medicaid Services (CMS), must have adequate emergency preparedness and disaster planning in place and readily available. These plans need to be reviewed annually and ASC staff should participate in educational forums that include practice of responses. Hazardous situations to an ASC can be of various types:

Natural Disasters such as tornadoes, hurricanes, earthquakes, extreme weather, wildfires, floods, volcanoes, or landslides.

Mechanical or Technological Failures consist of involvement with electrical, generators, gas or water supplies, building fires or floods, and HAZMAT or nuclear exposure that affects facility or causes structural damage.

Human Causes including biological or chemical terrorism, violent/armed intruder, and credible bomb threat or explosion.

As a sobering illustration, a 2010 publication, *the AHRQ Hospital Evacuation Decision Guide* (http://archive.ahrq.gov/prep/hospevacguide/), lists actual disasters encountered by healthcare facilities that included nuclear reactor incidents, earthquakes, nearby chemical plant explosion, bomb threat, hurricanes Katrina and Rita, wildfire, rising river, and a levy breach. Most of these occurrences resulted in evacuation from the medical facilities, even if that was not the initial pre-event anticipation or decision. Additionally, many of the disasters encountered provided no advance warning.[1]

Having well-written, disseminated, and rehearsed plans that are site-specific to your facilities' geographic location, physical layout, and unique needs will serve as the foundation of sound emergency preparedness.

The goals of emergency preparedness include:

1. Identify potential hazards or risks
2. Prevent loss of life
3. Mitigate trauma to the occupants of the ASC
4. Continue medical care to patients with as little interruption as possible
5. Minimize or prevent property damage.

Steps in the preparation of an effective emergency preparedness plan include:

1. Hazard identification and analysis: Identify potential hazards to the ASC, both internal and external, including geographic
2. Hazard mitigation: Outline steps to decrease the impact of the hazard before and after the event
3. Preparedness: Develop processes to meet the needs of patients, employees, and others on site at the ASC during an emergency event where essential services could break down as a result of a disaster
4. Response: Activities undertaken before, during, and after an emergency
5. Recovery: Activities designed to return the ASC to baseline
6. Plan coordination: The ASC must coordinate the Emergency Preparedness plan with state and local emergency response authorities
7. Testing/Evaluating/Updating: The ASC is required to conduct drills at least yearly, and have a written evaluation of each drill identifying problems that arose and a plan of correction. The Emergency Preparedness plan should then be updated to reflect the corrections.[2]

Perioperative Drill-Based Crisis Management, ed. Steven Butz. Published by Cambridge University Press. © Cambridge University Press 2016.

Detailed information and guidelines can be obtained on the CMS Emergency Preparedness website: www. cms.hhs.gov/SurveyCertEmergPrep/03_ HealthCareProviderGuidance.asp

Emergency operational plans (EOPs) for ASCs must include preparation for the incredible challenge of evacuation of the facility. Comprehensive resources for education and guidance in establishing your ASC's evacuation plan include the Harvard School of Public Health Emergency Preparedness and Response Exercise Program: Massachusetts Department of Public Health Hospital Evacuation Toolkit (see www. mass.gov), as well the AHRQ report.[3]

Key features of these are summarized:

1. In most emergencies a full evacuation is not required, but situations may arise that make it impossible to maintain a safe environment of care
2. The decision to evacuate is a difficult one that is likely to be made by a team of leaders after assessing safety threats and all possible alternatives[2]
3. Each institution should have a readily identifiable Incident Commander(IC).

The IC will need to understand and consider these integral components of any evacuation process in order to make optimal decisions.[2]

1. *Level of Evacuation*: can be dynamic depending on the nature, course, and severity of the event.[3] This would include sheltering-in-place, partial horizontal or vertical evacuations, or total evacuations
2. *Type of Evacuation* relates to priority of moving patient groups based on geography, available resources, or patient acuity
3. *Time Frame* depends on nature of threat and if any time allowed for preparation. This can be immediate, rapid, gradual, or prepare only
4. *Patient Prioritization* will take into consideration patients in immediate danger, ambulatory patients, those in the process of surgery or procedures, and those in various stages in recovery
5. *Pre-identified Assembly Points and Discharge Sites*
6. *Patient Tracking and Accompaniment of Pertinent Patient Information*
7. *Notification of Appropriate External Agencies.*

Evacuation goals and general principles to keep in mind[3]

1. Acknowledge that executing an evacuation is complex; care and processes will not always be optimal

2. Evacuation is an extremely labor-intensive process
3. Safety is the primary concern
4. Go for simplicity
5. Try to remain flexible and adaptable
6. Self-sufficiency is important; communication and direction from leaders may be difficult or impossible. Employees at every level must be knowledgeable in response and execution
7. You may need to evacuate before transportation, EMS, and receiving destinations are available
8. Try to keep patient care units together (Pre-op, ORs, PACU)
9. There may be difficult decisions and choices in which leaders and staff must focus on the "greatest good for the greatest number"
10. Full evacuation may be unavoidable but should generally be considered as a last resort.

The scenarios presented here are intended to illustrate situations that could result in the need for various response levels in an ASC in the middle of an operational day. There is no intent to either recommend or identify best practices or endorse any methodology. They are intended to be thought-provoking and idea-promoting with the result of stressing the need for continual attention to improving one's ASC's emergency responses. It is always recommended to use one's local area emergency manager as a resource for creating a facility plan.

Educational objectives

1. Understand the different types of hazards or disasters that your ASC could encounter
2. Become familiar with the goals of emergency preparedness
3. Become familiar with the steps of an emergency preparedness plan
4. Review and understand updated CMS requirements for ASCs
5. Become familiar with the different types of evacuation; how to implement and execute them
6. Understand the integral components that affect decision-making for evacuation plans.

Emergency preparedness and evacuation scenarios
Scenario 1: Gas leak

It is mid-morning in January at a freestanding ambulatory surgery center. Outside temperatures are in the

30s F (Ø, C). Two ORs have cases currently under way. You are the attending anesthesiologist and have just completed the induction of anesthesia with endotracheal intubation using rocuronium on your patient for breast reduction surgery. In an adjacent operating room there is a cataract surgery in progress under sedation. On the overhead paging system a voice announces, "All personnel please evacuate the building immediately."

Expected actions:

1. Confirm or verify the reason for the evacuation with the nursing director, charge nurse, or medical director
2. Identify who is the IC
3. Use available OR staff to move the patient from OR bed to a cart. Prepare to transport the patient with artificial manual breathing unit (AMBU) bag or transport circuit, oxygen cylinder(s), and any necessary drugs (total intravenous anesthetic (TIVA), reversal, and/or advanced cardiac life support (ACLS)). Use portable monitoring, if available. If not, prepare to transfer the code cart along with portable suction equipment to the identified assembly area to prepare for maintenance, emergence, and airway management
4. Instruct the other OR to stop surgery and prepare to transport the patient, likewise although simpler under monitored anesthesia care (MAC) anesthesia.

Scenario continued:

During construction at a building adjacent to the ASC, workmen accidentally severed the main gas line to the surgery center resulting in a major gas leak. The administrator has assumed the role of IC and has determined that full evacuation is necessary. She will:

1. Call 911 to obtain EMS and fire support
2. Notify surgery center security and local police to provide assistance, and ensure safety with crowd management and traffic flow
3. Notify receiving hospitals of incoming transfer patients.

The closest available shelter and assembly point is a medical office building located directly across a busy street.

Expected actions:

1. Due to the rapid nature of the evacuation and level of neuromuscular blockade, you will need to continue the anesthetic with TIVA until reaching the assembly point. Transport necessary equipment and supporting items for patient protection, safe anesthetic reversal, emergence, transfer, and recovery.
2. Have security and staff clear exit routes and assist in pushing carts through the snowy parking lot to the street. It is likely that they will have to secure the egress path by clearing any obstructions, negotiating any difficulties moving cart over curbs and ramps and across traffic
3. Support staff accompanies patient, anesthesia team, and surgeon with the necessary ACLS/code cart and portable suction equipment and any available portable monitoring
4. Make every effort to obtain and transfer patient personal health information, anesthetic records, and demographic information that will aid in communication with EMS, transfer facility, as well as family, friends or caregivers. Use any available methods including pen and paper.

Scenario continued:

The registration staff, at the direction of the IC, have stopped checking in patients, informed other patients and families of the leak, and instructed them to evacuate immediately as directed by arriving fire and police personnel.

The admitting staff gathers information regarding patient census that will aid in accounting for all patients and accompanying caregivers. The IC gathers information from team leaders and medical director regarding the staff census.

Expected actions:

1. Account for all individuals: patients, family, and staff
2. Use a check-in and check-out system at every transfer point: exiting the facility, arriving at the assembly point, discharge to caregiver, transfer, and arrival at receiving facility
3. Recover patients in the medical office building until EMS support arrives. Determine patients' disposition as stable for discharge or transfer to receiving facility
4. Appropriate patients may be discharged from a secondary discharge site to family or caregivers
5. Medical staff should accompany EMS transferring patients to receiving facility when feasible.

Scenario continued:

The fire department has arrived and assumed command. Unified command is established with the IC and the fire chief.

Expected actions:

1. Staff reports to ASC IC after evacuation of each area
2. Staff secures evacuated area from a safe zone to prevent people from re- entering the site
3. Staff, to the extent safely possible, turns off and unplugs all equipment, turns off all medical gases, and closes all doors and windows in the evacuated areas as they exit
4. IC notifies Emergency Management Director, Quality Assurance, and state Department of Health.

Scenario continued:

After initial assessment, it appears the facility will have to be closed for a week to allow for repairs.

Expected actions:

1. The IC will remain in communication with all personnel using the communication tree
2. Following repairs, the facility will need to be inspected by the State Department of Health and any other governing bodies
3. The "all clear" to resume normal operations is issued by the IC.

Scenario 2: Chemical spill

A large chemical spill has occurred in an equipment room in an ASC. The site is located midway between the preop and PACU areas in an area densely populated by staff and patients. Fumes emanating from the site are causing respiratory and eye irritation to those nearby. The Medical Director is on site and assumes the role of IC. It is mid-morning and five operating rooms have cases under way.

Expected actions:

1. Institute a horizontal partial evacuation from the preop and PACU, moving persons in immediate danger away from spill site to farthest side of facility on the same floor
2. Maintain appropriate level of supportive care and monitoring as feasible and the situation allows,

including supplemental oxygen, facemasks, and eye protection
3. Institute a "prepare to evacuate" response for the ORs in progress should the need arise
4. Contact 911 to call the local HAZMAT team and fire department, and give the exact location of the incident, the hazardous material involved, quantity of spill, and any ongoing reactions such as toxic fumes, corrosion, or fire
5. Attend to any staff exposures or injuries
6. Seal off or isolate the area if possible
7. Alert the rest of the facility by overhead paging, giving the exact location of the spill.

Scenario continued:

The HAZMAT team is en route. The administrator and Director of Nursing are also at the location. Several other employees have arrived at the site of the spill to serve as first responders until the fire department and HAZMAT arrive.

Expected actions:

1. IC compiles information as to the identity of the substance, along with pertinent information from the Material Safety Data Sheet (MSDS)
2. IC acts as liaison to the HAZMAT team and gathers/records information as the event evolves and will prepare a comprehensive incident report after the situation has been resolved
3. Staff having proper training should don designated personal protective equipment (including gowns, gloves, respiratory and eye protection) and use the content of the appropriate spill kit to effect as much containment as possible without endangering themselves.

Scenario continued:

Due to flammability potential of the chemical, the HAZMAT team orders a complete evacuation of the facility.

Expected actions:

1. IC changes the evacuation level for preop and PACU from horizontal to full evacuation of the facility
2. The facility ceases all current and further operations
3. IC directs ORs to now initiate full evacuation

4. Notify Emergency Medical Services to obtain the appropriate number and level of ambulances to provide support and transfer selected patients to receiving facilities

5. Notify security and/or local law enforcement to assist in securing the building and premises, as well as managing emergency vehicles, crowd control, and traffic

6. Notify receiving hospitals of incoming patients

7. The ORs, who were at a "prepare to evacuate" level, egress to the nearest exit avoiding the toxic area

8. Quickly complete or temporize surgical procedures using sutures, staples, occlusive, and other dressings

9. Assemble all appropriate equipment, drugs, and support. This includes sterile dressings and drapes, protection from the elements, oxygen cylinders, self-inflating rescue ventilation or transport bags, portable suction, code cart, drugs needed (TIVA and/or ACLS) to maintain anesthetics, and arrive at a selected safe zone or assembly point.

10. Staff escorts any remaining ambulatory patients, family, and visitors to safe zone and remains with them until they exit the premises

11. Team leaders account for all patients and staff

12. Appropriate patients are discharged to family or caregivers with instructions

13. Medical staff maintains stability of patients requiring transfer until EMS support arrives

14. Medical personnel accompany patients in transfer as needed, along with available pertinent medical information

15. IC notifies remaining appropriate agencies, including local Emergency Management Director, Department of Health, and insurers

16. Registration staff cancels scheduled patients.

Scenario continued:

The facility has been evacuated. Patients have been either discharged or transferred. The drill ends as fire department and HAZMAT clear the staff to enter and secure area, turning off all equipment and medical gases, closing all doors and windows, and completing initial clean-up and restoration. Once any damage to the facility has been repaired and the building has been inspected by the State Department of Health, the IC will give the "all clear" to resume normal operations.

Debriefing

1. Identify three things that went well with the scenario drill.

2. Identify three things that were difficult. How could they be improved?

3. Were any aspects of the drill so unsuccessful they should be reconsidered or reworked?

4. Did the staff understand their roles or did they require additional or intensive direction?

5. Was the entire team able to participate in the scenario to optimize simulation of a real-life drill?

6. Would it be useful to have each participant's role outlined on cards as an aid during any future drills?

7. Did participants actually perform the required actions?

8. Did the drill test an evacuation route to evaluate its accessibility?

9. Did the drill test pertinent phone numbers to ensure accurate communication?

10. Were any outside agencies, first responders, law enforcement, or building security invited to attend? If not, would this be helpful in future drills?

11. Did the participants feel free to openly ask questions and offer suggestions?

Discussion

The first step in creating, or refining, an emergency preparedness ("disaster") plan for one's ASC should be acknowledging the possibility and probability of what types of event could result in severe hardship in maintaining a safe level of care. Whether causation is natural or man-made, it is recommended that plans begin with Pre-Disaster Risk Assessments that identify and anticipate:

1. Specific disasters that could affect vulnerable aspects of the ASC's structural integrity, most importantly heating, ventilation, and air-conditioning (HVAC), water, and electricity where compromise would critically hamper normal operations

2. Life-threatening or emergency situations, such as chemical or biological contamination, fire, or explosion/bomb threat, that could pose an imminent threat to patients, employees and others

3. Challenges the ASC would face in having to disrupt care and move patients around or out of the facility,

including transfer to predetermined outlying medical facilities or hospitals

4. Any measures that would mitigate or minimize further damage to equipment, building, or property

5. Recovery measures needed to restore the facility and employees to its usual state or "new normal". This should include some aspect of critical incident stress debriefing and employee support

6. A Business Impact Analysis if the critical business process would be interrupted for a significant length of time. [1,4]

Following that assessment, specific plans and documents should be generated and disseminated that include an authority chain. This identifies a decision-making administrator or manager, an *IC* (and alternates), as well as a list of all employees (with contact numbers) and in which roles they can serve.

A *communication roster* should be readily available that includes numbers for: Police, fire, EMS, security, all utilities, building management, County Office of Emergency Management, receiving hospitals for patient transfers, IT resources, and insurance companies. [4]

If the threat level is sufficient to consider triggering an evacuation, the administrators and IC need to have an awareness of factors that enter into a decision-making tree. This may aid in choosing the level of evacuation that would meet the needs of the situation, acknowledging that the event could be dynamic and original plans could change. No single formula or algorithm could possibly capture all the nuances or iterations one may encounter, [1] but familiarity with the following concepts may help clarify an uncertain situation.

Levels of evacuation: Reflect increasing scope and severity[3]

Shelter-in-place:

1. Requires cessation of all routine activities

2. No further patients should be admitted; no new procedures started

3. Typically, patients, staff, and visitors remain where they are with certain mitigations such as closing doors, windows and blinds, relocating away from windows to a more central area.

Horizontal evacuation:

1. Moving patients in immediate danger away from the threat to an area of refuge: an adjacent smoke/fire zone or the opposite side of building

2. Usually the fastest option

3. Facilitates the simplest re-entry process.

Vertical evacuation:

1. The complete evacuation of a specific floor in a building

2. Usually evacuate toward the ground level at least two floors below.

Total evacuation:

1. Usually used as a last resort

2. Involves complete evacuation of facility.

Type of evacuation: Determines priority for moving group of patients

Geographic model:

1. Evacuate the areas of greatest risk or select individual units.

Resource model:

1. Utilize resources in the most efficient manner

2. Patient evacuation priority is linked to resource availability.

Acuity model:

1. Evacuate according to acuity such that the most mobile patients are evacuated first

2. Ensure the greatest good for the greatest number

3. This would mean that anesthetized patients requiring continued surgical and anesthetic support may be evacuated last and not until absolutely necessary. This could allow time for the appropriate transport vehicles and EMS support.

Note that it is possible that portions of each of these models could be used concurrently depending on the dynamics of the situation. [3]

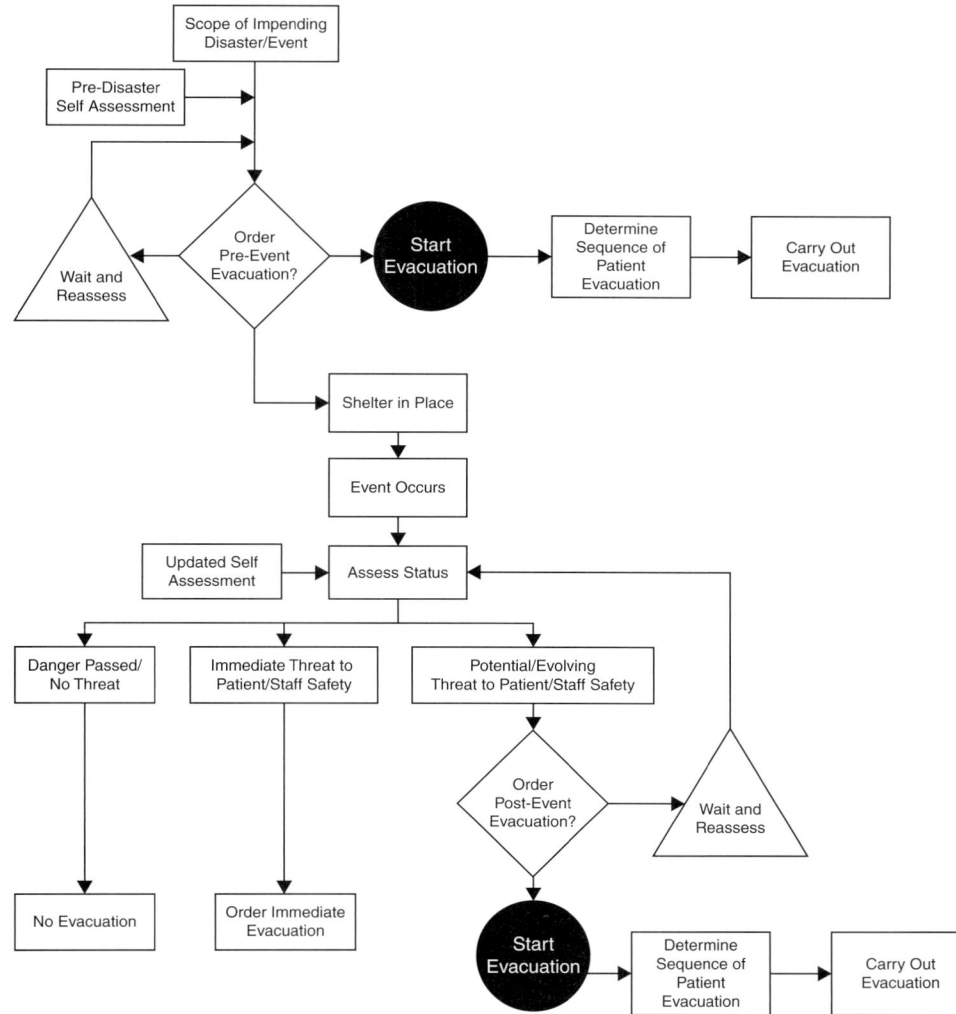

Figure 10.1
Advanced warning event evacuation decisions. Reprinted from AHRQ Publication No. 10-0009, May 2010

Evacuation time frames[1]

With an *impending event* where the ASC environment is not yet compromised (*Advanced Warning Event*), a decision must be made whether to preemptively evacuate or to shelter-in-place (Figure 10.1).

This decision should take into consideration:

1. The nature of the event, along with the expected duration, severity, and the area(s) impacted
2. The anticipated effect on the structure or key resources needed to maintain care and therefore, patient safety. Try to ascertain whether an impending disaster would place patients and staff at unacceptable risk

3. The possibility that evacuation after the event would be increasingly dangerous or impossible.

If an event or disaster has already occurred (*No Advanced Warning Event*), the determination will have to be made as to whether the ASC can continue to provide appropriate level of care to patients. If compromised, decide to institute a shelter-in-place, a partial evacuation, or a full evacuation (Figure 10.2).

It is also important to distinguish between a *type of event* that could precipitate consideration of an evacuation (natural disaster, technological hazard, explosion) and the *actual reason* that makes an evacuation

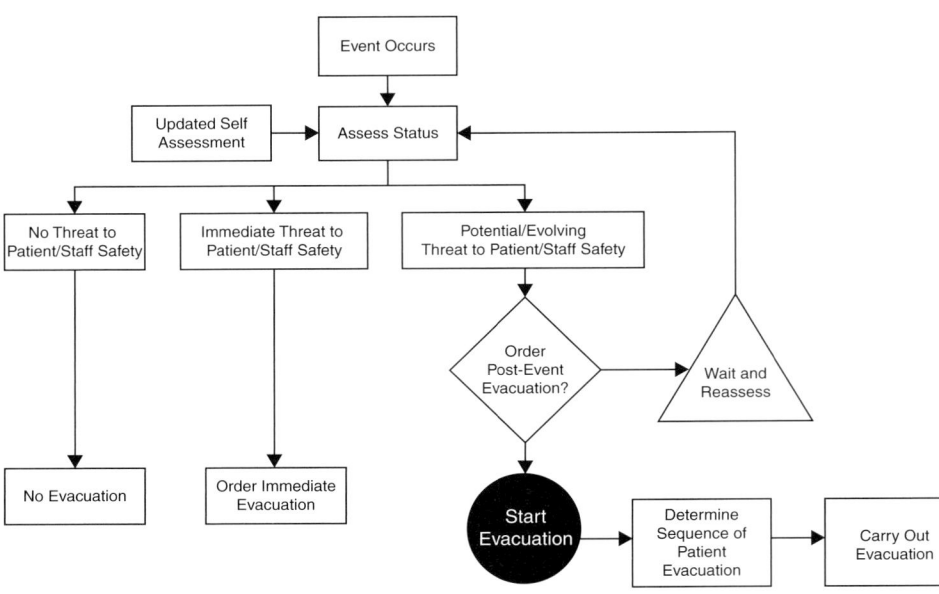

Figure 10.2 No advanced warning event evacuation decisions. Reprinted from AHRQ Publication No. 10-0009, May 2010

necessary (structural damage, air quality contamination, utility loss).

Assembly point(s) and discharge sites

Locations surrounding the facility need to be identified as potential safe zones.

Assembly Points can be patient care sites where it is possible to provide basic care and await transfer or be deemed ready for discharge. Supplies, equipment, and staff would be concentrated there. Patients would be accounted for and managed.

Discharge Sites can be areas where patients wait for family or friends to pick them up. If possible, locate this away from the Assembly Point to optimize traffic flow and reduce congestion. Patients would be accounted for and given any necessary supplies and instructions.

Both of these could be affected by environmental variables or hazardous conditions. Nearby locations should be identified and confirmed in the ASC's disaster plan as willing to help provide shelter and support while awaiting definitive BLS/ACLS ambulance transport and transfer.

Patient tracking and medical information transfer

A system to keep track of all patients during an emergency evacuation is imperative. This may resort to a basic paper-based system that "checks-in" and "checks-out" patients at various points throughout the

process.[3] Admitting can provide a patient census to help with accountability.

These would ideally include:

1. Leaving the patient care unit (preop, intra-op, PACU)
2. Arrival at Assembly Point or Discharge Site
3. Leaving the Assembly Point or Discharge Site
4. Arriving at a staging area to await transfer
5. Leaving the staging area at transfer
6. Arrival at the destination/receiving hospital.

Medical records, personal health information, and pertinent surgical/anesthetic notes should accompany transfer patients as the situation allows.

Whether sheltering-in-place or carrying out a full evacuation, an ASC will need a comprehensive plan that takes into consideration the individual physical plant; number of patients and their varying medical acuity; available personnel and resources; entry and egress points; closest usable shelter or assembly point(s); proximity of local fire, police, and EMS to provide assistance, security, and transportation; and identifiable destinations for patient transfer.

At any one time during the operational day in an ASC, many patients in the pre- and postoperative units will be medically stable and able to be moved easily by self-ambulation, help from family members, wheelchairs, or carts with little or no sophisticated medical equipment necessary should the need arise.

The challenge arises in the management of patients that are undergoing operative procedures. Depending on the surgical services that make up the center and the number of operating rooms, a certain percentage of patients might be expected to be under monitored anesthesia care (MAC) anesthesia for relatively peripheral procedures such as ophthalmologic or orthopedic. These could be managed by sterile covers to operative sites, minimal supportive care, and transfer horizontally to safer area or exit by cart or wheelchair.

But should any, or the majority, of procedures fall under those that typically require general anesthesia and the operation is aborted or not completed, the patient may need to remain anesthetized with airway management for an extended time period. Planning exercises should take into account equipment (oxygen tanks, self-inflating rescue-breathing or transfer bags, portable suction, adjunct airways items, monitors), drugs (TIVA and ACLS), and personnel needed to transfer horizontally or exit the building. This needs to include an estimate of the number of BLS or ACLS support vehicles (communicated in the initial 911 call) that would be required for transfer to another facility for completion of operation and safe emergence from anesthesia.

If EMS transfer is needed, the decision will need to take into account whether there is an assembly point or location that will be utilized first (including outdoors) where patients could then be loaded into vehicles.[1] There could very possibly be a need for medical personnel (surgeons, anesthesia providers, and/or nurses) to accompany patients with as much medical record and supportive information as time and the situation allow.

CMS recently amended their regulations for dealing with disaster preparedness in ASCs. This updated document (regulation 416.54) is included for review.[2] The details outlined in the conditions for coverage encompass the following basic elements:

1. Emergency plans
2. Policies and procedures
3. Communication plan
4. Training and testing.

On a practical level, it is difficult to execute drills that simulate evacuations. A possible starting place for this type of education could be in-service presentations followed by table-top discussions of scenarios.

This author has used the "captive audience approach" of surgeons and staff during the OR work day to consider and discuss exactly what it would take to safely evacuate the present patients in a "drop-and-go" situation, such as the gas leak. This has resulted in surgeons spelling out what they would need for temporary closure, packing, sterile dressings, and cover to exit the OR to the outside environment. The circulator and scrub techs engage in what support they would provide and roles they would play. The anesthesiologist and CRNA or AA devise plans of what drugs and equipment they would take; if, how, and when they would emerge and manage airway; as well as how they would support patients if no EMS and ambulance was readily available. Doing this on multiple and varying days with different surgical services can cover all members of the ASC staff and generate confidence in managing critical situations.

Moving to consideration of the entire ASC, it could be helpful to intermittently and repeatedly take "snapshots" of the different units at varying times and days and then analyze those "moments in time" to estimate what level of support and resources would be needed to evacuate the premises quickly:

1. How many bays are occupied in preop and PACU?
2. Are there family members present? Can they help or will they need support to evacuate also?
3. What is the nurse–patient ratio at that moment?
4. Which other ancillary staff are present and what roles could they play?
5. Which egresses are available and who uses which way?
6. Could you easily access patients' shoes, outerwear, and possessions or would this be time prohibitive? What alternatives are available to protect patients in the current outside environment?
7. How many ORs are being utilized at the moment and how many of these patients are under general anesthesia such that they will need EMS ambulances?
8. This walk-though exercise can prove enlightening for medical directors, managers, and administrators in evaluating their present emergency preparedness plans
9. Lastly, where, how far away, and what type of building is closest to the ASC that could be used to provide shelter if needed? Consider meeting with the occupants to ascertain their willingness, and the logistics needed, to occupy that space temporarily while awaiting outside support. Document that agreement in your plan.

A well-designed emergency preparedness plan coupled with education, implementation, and practice can fulfill your ASC's specific accreditation standards, fulfill CMS requirements, and enhance your staff's competency and confidence, all with the intent of optimizing your ASC's outcomes in the event of any type of disaster.

Checklist for ASC emergency preparedness plans

1. The facility has a specifically developed written emergency preparedness plan(s)
2. The plan is developed by a designated committee that identifies an individual in charge of oversight
3. The plan attempts to identify and take into account all hazards specific to the ASC location
4. The plan indicates the date of last review and is continually updated with respect to recent changes in staff, contact information, transfer agreements, and facility floor plans
5. The plan is easily accessible in multiple locations which are known to staff, administration, management, security, and possibly local first responders
6. The plan includes floor plans, location of emergency exits, smoke barriers, and main utility shut-offs
7. The plan is annually reviewed and documented by all employees in an in-service educational session or table-top discussion led by a facilitator
8. The plan is included and documented as part of new employee orientation and training
9. Employees are aware of the various roles in which they may be called to serve or execute
10. The facility conducts and documents at least two drills of the plan, not including fire drills, within each 12-month period
11. Each drill is followed by a debriefing, written evaluation, identification of any problems with plan(s) of correction, and maintains documentation of such
12. The plan includes a policy for critical incident stress debriefing
13. The plan designates an information or media spokesperson and media area so as not to interfere with continued operations of the ASC or evacuations in progress

14. The plan complies with local, state, and federal requirements
15. The plan can be communicated to local, county, and state agencies and authorities
16. The plan outlines measures to restore the facility and business to pre-disaster levels.

Checklist for ASC evacuation plan

1. The plan identifies an official(s) vested with the authority to initiate a partial or full evacuation. This could be dynamic depending on the acuity and severity of the event
2. The plan designates a chain of command that includes an on-site leader(s) to function as IC
3. The plan includes preferred communication methods such as an automated emergency notification system, overhead paging, email, or texting to notify appropriate personnel of decision to evacuate
4. The plan identifies chosen locations for assembly points, secondary sites for shelter, discharge site locations, and EMS pick-up/transfer sites. Under IC jurisdiction, these can be dynamic
5. The plan identifies egress routes. These can be evaluated or prioritized on the basis of potential ease or difficulty with cart transfer or ambulation. This could be dynamic
6. The plan includes a call list for police, fire, EMS, local and state emergency management agencies, utilities, HAZMAT, and medical gas suppliers; reviewed and updated periodically
7. The plan includes an IC phone roster of administration, medical staff, and employees; reviewed and updated periodically
8. The facility has a plan for sheltering-in-place
9. The facility has a valid transfer agreement with a receiving hospital or facility that has an equivalent or greater level of service
10. The facility has a transportation plan that accommodates and supports both basic and advanced EMS along with a back-up plan if primary transportation services are not available
11. The plan includes a system to track location of patients, staff, visitors, and volunteers during and after the evacuation
12. The plan includes a method to handle patient identification, medical records, and pertinent

health information during evacuation, transfer, and receivership.

References

1. Zane R, Biddinger P, Hassol A, Rich T, Gerber J, DeAngelis J. Hospital evacuation decision guide. (Prepared under Contract No. 290-20-0600-011.) AHRQ Publication No. 10-0009. Rockville, MD: Agency for Healthcare Research and Quality. May 2010. http://archive.ahrq.gov/prep/hospevacguide/ (accessed January 4, 2015).
2. CMS.gov Health Care Provider Guidance Survey & Certification Emergency Preparedness http://www.cms.hhs.gov/SurveyCertEmergPrep/03_HealthCareProviderGuidance.asp#TopOfPage (accessed January 5, 2015).
3. Harvard School of Public Health Emergency Preparedness and Response Exercise Program: II. Hospital Evacuation Planning Guide http://www.mass.gov/eohhs/docs/dph/emergency-prep/hospital-evacuation-toolkit/planning-guide.pdf (accessed January 4, 2015).
4. Sibulsky, M. AAAHC Update: Writing a disaster plan for your ASC http://ortoday.com/aaahc-update-writing-a-disaster-plan-for-your-asc/ (accessed December 29, 2014).

Index